T.

Tracheotomy Management

A Multidisciplinary Approach

Tracheotomy Management

A Multidisciplinary Approach

Edited by

Peggy A. Seidman MD FAAP
Clinical Associate Professor,
Departments of Anesthesiology and Pediatrics
Division Chief Pediatric Anesthesiology
SUNY at Stony Brook School of Medicine
Stony Brook, NY USA

David Goldenberg MD FACS
Professor of Surgery and Oncology
Director of Head and Neck Surgery
Pennsylvania State University College of Medicine
Hershey, PA USA

Elizabeth H. Sinz MD
Professor of Anesthesiology, Critical Care Medicine and Neurosurgery and
Associate Dean of Clinical Simulation
Pennsylvania State University College of Medicine
Hershey, PA USA

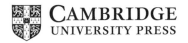

CAMBRIDGE
UNIVERSITY PRESS

CAMBRIDGE UNIVERSITY PRESS
Cambridge, New York, Melbourne, Madrid, Cape Town,
Singapore, São Paulo, Delhi, Tokyo, Mexico City

Cambridge University Press
The Edinburgh Building, Cambridge CB2 8RU, UK

Published in the United States of America by Cambridge University Press,
New York

www.cambridge.org
Information on this title: www.cambridge.org/9780521196918

© Cambridge University Press 2011

First published 2011

Printed in the United Kingdom at the University Press, Cambridge

A catalog record for this publication is available from the British Library

Library of Congress Cataloging in Publication data
Tracheotomy management : a multidisciplinary approach / edited by Peggy A. Seidman, Elizabeth H. Sinz,
David Goldenberg.
    p. ; cm.
Includes bibliographical references and index.
ISBN 978-0-521-19691-8 (pbk.)
1. Tracheotomy – Patients – Care.   2. Trachea – Surgery.   I. Seidman, Peggy A., 1959–   II. Sinz,
Elizabeth.   III. Goldenberg, David, 1962–
[DNLM: 1. Tracheotomy – methods.   2. Trachea – surgery.   3. Tracheal Diseases – surgery. WF 490]
RF517.T733   2011
617.5'33–dc23

                                                                                                    2011023011

ISBN 978 0 521 19691 8 Paperback

Contents

Preface   page vii
List of contributors   viii
Acknowledgements   xii

Introduction: the history of tracheotomy 1
Zahra Karparvar and David Goldenberg

1. **Anatomy of the anterior and lateral neck** 12
Elliot Regenbogen

2. **Elective surgical tracheotomy in the adult** 28
Yvonne Tsui, Michael Ondik, and David Goldenberg

3. **Percutaneous tracheotomy** 39
Garret Choby, Dmitri Bezinover, and David Goldenberg

4. **Emergency surgical airways** 51
Leonard Pott and Scott Goldstein

5. **Congenital, embryological, and anatomic variations, and their association with pediatric tracheotomy** 63
Elliot Regenbogen

6. **Pediatric tracheotomy** 72
Robert Yellon, Raymond Maguire, and Jay B. Tuchman

7. **Laryngotracheal reconstruction: surgical management of pediatric airway stenosis** 87
Diego Preciado, Sophie R. Pestieau, and Ira Todd Cohen

8. **Timing of tracheotomy for intubated patients** 99
Alison Wilson, Elias B. Rizk, Kimberly E. Fenton, Thomas K. Lee, and Elizabeth H. Sinz

9. **Intensive care unit tracheotomy care** 117
Shaji Poovathoor, Eric Posner, James Vosswinkel, and Peggy A. Seidman

10. **Complications of tracheotomy** 126
Steven L. Orebaugh

11. **Airway manipulation with tracheotomy** 134
Daryn H. Moller, Slawomir Oleszak, and Ghassan J. Samara

12. **Tracheotomy equipment** 146
Dana Stauffer, John Stene, and Joanne Stene

13. **Care of the patient with a tracheotomy** 165
Margaret Wojnar and Jonathan D. McGinn

14. **Tracheotomy education for home care** 180
Jodie E. Landis, Michael K. Hurst, and Brian W. Grose

Index   195

v

Preface

When confronted with a challenging clinical problem, help can frequently be found in textbooks or a search of the literature. Unfortunately, for questions about tracheotomies, the resources were either parceled in multiple diverse sources or buried in the lore of different subspecialties. A wide range of healthcare providers treat patients with a surgical airway and a mix of different providers must be ready to obtain or manage a surgical airway in an emergency. With the increasing prevalence of patients with tracheotomies, a book written from a concensus approach by the different healthcare providers encountering them was needed. The result is this text, useful when caring for anyone with a surgical airway.

This book provides a concise but comprehensive summary of current treatments and techniques. In each chapter, the authors are drawn from different specialties to provide a comprehensive view of each topic covered. Sample clinical cases are described to provide context. While each chapter can be used independently for specific topics, the book also serves as a complete resource for anyone confronted with uncommon clinical situations that can arise in people with surgical airways.

The history of tracheotomy has been steeped in controversy since its inception; however, the past century has seen many advances. Although evidence-based recommendations are given when possible, there is still more to learn. It is our hope that this text will improve healthcare providers' undertanding and ability to take care of the tracheotomized patient.

The Editors:
Peggy Seidman
David Goldenberg
Elizabeth Sinz

Contributors

Dmitri Bezinover MD, PhD
Assistant Professor of Anesthesiology
Department of Anesthesiology
Pennsylvania State University College
of Medicine
The Penn State Milton S. Hershey
Medical Center
Hershey, PA USA

Ira Todd Cohen MD, MEd, FAAP
Professor of Anesthesiology and Pediatrics
Division of Anesthesiology and Pain Medicine
The George Washington University
Children's National Medical Center
Washington, DC, USA

Garret Choby MD
Division of Otolaryngology-Head and Neck
Surgery
Pennsylvania State University College
of Medicine
The Penn State Milton S. Hershey Medical
Center
Hershey, PA USA

Kimberly E. Fenton MD, FAAP
Associate Professor of Pediatrics
Division of Critical Care Medicine
SUNY at Stony Brook School of Medicine
Stony Brook, NY USA

David Goldenberg MD, FACS
Professor of Surgery and Oncology
Director of Head and Neck Surgery
Division of Otolaryngology-Head and Neck
Surgery
Pennsylvania State University College
of Medicine
The Penn State Milton S. Hershey Medical
Center
Hershey, PA USA

Scott Goldstein DO
Assistant Professor of Emergency Medicine
Department of Emergency Medicine
Pennsylvania State University College of
Medicine
The Penn State Milton S. Hershey Medical
Center
Hershey, PA USA

Brian W. Grose MD
Assistant Professor of Anesthesia
Vice Chair for Clinical Operations
West Virginia University School of
Medicine
Morgantown, WV USA

Michael K. Hurst DDS, MD
Associate Professor of Otolaryngology
Department of Otolaryngology – Head and
Neck Surgery
West Virginia University School
of Medicine
Morgantown, WV USA

Zara Karparvar MD
Pennsylvania State University College of
Medicine
The Penn State Milton S. Hershey Medical
Center
Hershey, PA USA

Jodie E. Landis MS, CCC-SLP
Speech Language Pathologist
Morgantown, WV USA

Thomas K. Lee MD
Associate Professor of Surgery and
Pediatrics Chief, Pediatric Surgery
Department of Pediatric Surgery
SUNY at Stony Brook School of Medicine
Stony Brook, NY USA

Jonathan D. McGinn MD

Associate Professor of Surgery Division of
Otolaryngology – Head and Neck Surgery
Pennsylvania State University College of
Medicine
The Penn State Milton S. Hershey Medical
Center
Hershey, PA USA

Raymond Maguire DO

Assistant Professor of Otolaryngology
Division of Pediatric Otolaryngology
Children's Hospital of Pittsburgh of
UPMC
University of Pittsburgh School of Medicine
Pittsburgh, PA USA

Daryn H. Moller MD

Associate Professor of Anesthesiology
Department of Anesthesiology
Division Chief, General/Vascular/Trauma
Anesthesia
SUNY at Stony Brook School of Medicine
Stony Brook, NY USA

Slawomir Oleszak MD

Assistant Professor of Anesthesiology
Department of Anesthesiology
SUNY at Stony Brook School of Medicine
Stony Brook, NY USA

Michael Ondik MD

Division of Otolaryngology-Head and Neck
Surgery Pennsylvania State University
College of Medicine
The Penn State Milton S. Hershey Medical
Center
Hershey, PA USA

Steven L. Orebaugh MD

Associate Professor of Anesthesiology and
Critical Care Medicine Department of
Anesthesiology
University of Pittsburgh School
of Medicine
UPMC-Southside/Mercy
Pittsburgh, PA USA

Sophie R. Pestieau MD

Assistant Professor of Anesthesiology and
Pediatrics Division of Anesthesiology and
Pain Medicine
The George Washington University
Children's National Medical Center
Washington, DC, USA

Shaji Poovathoor MD

Assistant Professor of Clinical
Anesthesiology and Critical Care Medicine
Department of Anesthesiology
SUNY at Stony Brook School of Medicine
Stony Brook, NY USA

Eric Posner MD

Clinical Assistant Professor of
Anesthesiology,
SUNY at Stony Brook School of Medicine
Stony Brook, NY USA

Leonard Pott MBBCh FCA(SA)

Associate Professor of Anesthesiology and
Emergency Medicine Department of
Anesthesiology
Pennsylvania State University College
of Medicine
The Penn State Milton S. Hershey
Medical Center
Hershey, PA USA

Diego Preciado MD, PhD

Assistant Professor of Surgery and
Pediatrics Division Pediatric
Otolaryngology – Head and Neck
Surgery
The George Washington University
Children's National Medical Center
Washington, DC, USA

Elliot Regenbogen MD

Assistant Professor of Surgery Division
Otolaryngology, Head and Neck Surgery
SUNY at Stony Brook School
of Medicine
Stony Brook, NY USA

Elias B. Rizk MD
Chief Resident Department of Neurosurgery
Pennsylvania State University College of
Medicine
The Penn State Milton S. Hershey Medical
Center
Hershey, PA USA

Ghassan J. Samara MD, FACS
Associate Professor of Surgery Director of
Rhinology, Research
Division of Otolaryngology, Head and Neck
Surgery
SUNY at Stony Brook School of Medicine
Stony Brook, NY USA

Peggy A. Seidman MD, FAAP
Clinical Associate Professor,
Departments of Anethesiology and Pediatrics
Division Chief Pediatric Anesthesiology
SUNY at Stony Brook School
of Medicine
Stony Brook, NY USA

Elizabeth H. Sinz MD
Professor of Anesthesiology, Critical Care
Medicine and Neurosurgery and
Associate Dean of Clinical Simulation
Departments of Anesthesiology and
Neurosurgery
Pennsylvania State University College of
Medicine
The Penn State Milton S. Hershey Medical
Center
Hershey, PA USA

Dana Stauffer MS, RRT-NPS
Manager, Respiratory Care and Pulmonary
Diagnostics
The Penn State Milton S. Hershey Medical
Center
Hershey, PA USA

Joanne Stene BS, RN, RRT
Department of Nursing Derry Township
School District
Hershey, PA USA

John Stene MD, PhD
Professor of Anesthesiology and
Neurosurgery Departments of
Anesthesiology and Neurosurgery
Pennsylvania State University College of
Medicine
The Penn State Milton S. Hershey Medical
Center
Hershey, PA USA

Jay B. Tuchman MD, FAAP
Assistant Professor of Anesthesiology
Department of Anesthesiology
Children's Hospital of Pittsburgh
University of Pittsburgh School
of Medicine
Pittsburgh, PA USA

Yvonne Tsui MD
Division of Otolaryngology-Head
and Neck Surgery
Pennsylvania State University College of
Medicine
The Penn State Milton S. Hershey Medical
Center
Hershey, PA USA

James Vosswinkel MD
Assistant Professor
Department of Surgery
Director of Surgical Intensive
Care Unit
SUNY at Stony Brook School
of Medicine
Stony Brook, NY USA

Alison Wilson MD
Associate Professor of Surgery
Director, Jon Michael Moore Trauma
Center
Chief, Trauma, Emergency Surgery and
Surgical Critical Care
Department of Surgery West Virginia
University School of Medicine
Morgantown, WV USA

Margaret Wojnar MD
Professor of Medicine Division Pulmonary,
Allergy and Critical Care Medicine
Pennsylvania State University College of
Medicine
The Penn State Milton S. Hershey Medical
Center
Hershey, PA USA

Robert Yellon MD
Professor of Otolaryngology Division of
Pediatric Otolaryngology
Children's Hospital of Pittsburgh
of UPMC
University of Pittsburgh School of Medicine
Pittsburgh, PA USA

Acknowledgements

We can only reach for the stars by standing on shoulders of those before us. I am only where I am with the help of many teachers and colleagues who gave me time, advice and support. To my children Eli and Samuel, you will always be the most important work I ever produced.

Peggy Seidman

My deepest gratitude to my parents for their support, to my wife, Renee, who is an invaluable partner in my life, and to my beloved children Michael, Ellie, and Dana.

David Goldenberg

I have been fortunate to have many good teachers and a few great mentors. All have given me their time, patience, and what little wisdom I possess. Thanks to my husband, David, for giving me uninterrupted time to complete this book, and to my daughters, Claire, Caroline, and Kate who distracted me enough to stop working and digest the material.

Lisa Sinz

Introduction: the history of tracheotomy

Zahra Karparvar and David Goldenberg

Case presentation

In 1799, Elisha Cullen Dick, a former pupil of Benjamin Rush, was called to help attend to George Washington. Dr. Dick and two other physicians used copious bleeding in addition to other medical procedures. Dr. Dick suggested that a tracheotomy be performed to relieve the General's obstructed airway. This suggestion was overruled and Washington died of obstruction from an upper airway infection.

Introduction

Tracheotomy is one of the oldest surgical procedures described, with written descriptions dating back to ancient Egypt and India. Its safety and necessity have been controversial for centuries. The indications and techniques for tracheotomy have changed and expanded over time. Today, due to advances in intensive care medicine and the widespread use of mechanical ventilation, tracheotomy is one of the most commonly performed surgical procedures. Owing to its increased prevalence, it is encountered on a regular basis by physicians in all fields of medicine.

The extensive history of tracheotomy can best be divided into five periods.

The period of legend (3100 BC to AD 1546)

It is impossible to know exactly when the first tracheotomy was attempted, but there is evidence from hieroglyph slabs belonging to King Djer in Abydos and King Aha in Saqqara that tracheotomy was performed in ancient Egypt at about 3100 BC [1]. Tracheotomy is also mentioned in the Rig Veda, a sacred book of Hindu medicine written between 2000 and 1000 BC. These writings describe "the bountiful one who without ligature, can cause the windpipe to reunite when the cervical cartilages are cut across, provided that they are not entirely severed" [2]. The Ebers Papyrus, an ancient medical reference from 1550 BC, refers to opening the windpipe through a neck incision [3] and in the eighth century BC Homer referred to an operation to relieve choking persons by cutting the trachea [4]. In the fourth century BC, Alexander the Great is said to have saved the life of a soldier who was choking from a bone lodged in his throat by "puncturing his trachea" with the point of his sword [4].

The first elective tracheotomy is credited to Asclepiades of Bithynia in AD 100 [3]. This operation was described by the renowned physician Claudius Galen in AD 131 [5] who also contributed to the understanding of the tracheotomy by describing the anatomy of the head

Tracheotomy Management: A Multidisciplinary Approach, ed. Peggy A. Seidman,
David Goldenberg and Elizabeth H. Sinz. Published by Cambridge University Press.
© Cambridge University Press 2011.

and neck [6]. In the same century, Aretaeus in his book, *The Therapeutics of Acute Diseases*, confirmed the work done by Asclepiades of Bithynia on the subject of tracheotomy, but he condemned it on the grounds that "cartilage wounds do not heal" [7]. Later, in the fifth century AD, *Caelius Aurelianus* condemned the operation and stated, "Laryngotomia is a futile and irresponsible idea set forth by Asclepiades" [8]. Albucasis (936–1013) contributed to the history of tracheotomy by suturing a tracheal wound and demonstrating its ability to heal in a servant girl who had tried to commit suicide by cutting her throat [9,10].

The Dark Ages (fifth to fifteenth centuries AD) eclipsed the world of science and medicine with scarce mention of any type of surgery until the fifteenth century. It is interesting to note that many authors of this period described tracheotomy in detail, but they denied performing the operation themselves. References were made to tracheotomy, but the operation was officially considered both useless and dangerous due to the high risk of wound infection and a belief that cartilage rings could not heal.

The period of fear (AD 1546–1833)

The period between 1546 and 1833 marks the "period of fear" in the history of tracheotomy. During this era the procedure was considered irresponsible and barbaric, and only 28 successful tracheotomies were recorded in the literature [11]. In Bologna, Rolandi used tracheotomy to alleviate obstruction caused by laryngeal abscess [12]. In 1546, Antonio Musa Brasavola is quoted as saying "When there is no other possibility, in angina, of admitting air to the heart, we must incise the larynx below the abscess." This account describes the use of tracheotomy to obtain an emergency airway in Ludwig's angina (submental space abscess) [6,13] and although there are some records of tracheotomy for the treatment of Ludwig's angina by Saliceto and Paré in France [12], this was not the treatment of choice by anyone's standards at that time [6].

An Italian anatomist, Fabricius ab Aquapendente (1537–1619) also described the use of tracheotomy to bypass an obstruction of the airway, writing, "The terrified surgeons of our times have not dared to exercise this surgery and I also have never performed it; it is a scandal" [6]. Later though, he modified his feelings and successfully performed tracheotomies to relieve laryngeal obstruction due to foreign bodies. He used a vertical incision and a cannula with flanges. His pupil Casserius, introduced the curved cannula with stay tapes to hold it in position, but unfortunately this improvement in tube shape was quickly forgotten, and the straight tracheotomy tube remained in use for many years [7]. In 1590, Sanctorius used a trocar and cannula with a short, straight tube, the tip of which was placed against the tracheoesophageal wall and the cannula left in place for 3 days [14].

By the early 1600s, tracheotomy was considered acceptable for acute upper airway obstruction caused by foreign body ingestion, aspiration, and infection [7]. During the diphtheria epidemic in Naples, Severigno used tracheotomy as a symptomatic treatment (Julius Casserius 1599). Records from 1620 indicate that Nicholas Habicot of Paris did four successful tracheotomies leading him to suggest that the operation be used for inflammatory conditions of the larynx [15]. Interestingly, one of his tracheotomies was used to relieve the respiratory obstruction caused by the pressure of gold coins in the esophagus swallowed by a 14-year-old boy to protect his possessions from theft. The bag of coins became lodged in his esophagus impinging on his airway. Habicot used a novel tracheotomy tube that was flatter than usual to prevent pressure necrosis in the surrounding tissue [15]. In 1650, a renowned surgical pathologist named Theophilus Bonetus recommended the use

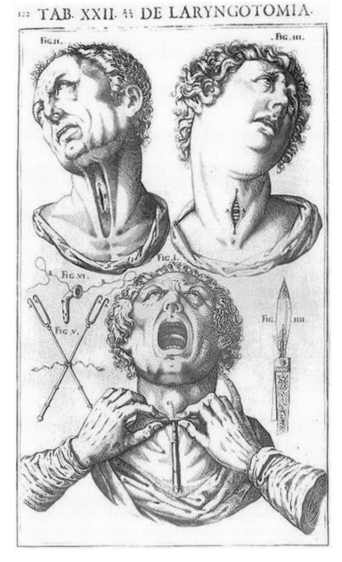

Figure 1 Julius Casserius – Tracheotomy- *Tabulae Anatomicae* 1601.

of a tracheotomy for a 7-year-old child who had aspirated a piece of bone. This suggestion was rejected by the internist in accordance with the times and the child died [16].

There were other instances of physicians using tracheotomy for the symptomatic relief of respiratory infections. Renaus Moreau suggested its use in mumps [7], recommending that the procedure be performed with the patient in the supine position, a recommendation that was ignored for nearly 200 years [17]. In 1765, Francis Home, a Scottish physician, recommended the use of tracheotomy to alleviate respiratory compromise in children suffering from croup [18] (called cynanche trachealis in the United States, with the direct Greek translation meaning dog-like choking). Despite the high prevalence of cases in the United States and Great Britain, fear and mistrust of the procedure prevented prevalent therapeutic use [18]. Professor Wendt of Erlangen, in 1760, described tracheotomy in a young patient via opening the trachea by dividing the first three rings and separating edges of the wound with blunt hooks [19]. In 1770, William Buchan's handbook for physicians devoted a chapter to the management of drowning patients, one of which was on opening the trachea. This material originated from the *Memoire sur la bronchotomie*, a text written by Louis who also advocated the use of tracheotomy for the extraction of foreign objects, which led to criticism from other practitioners.

The New World was heavily influenced by the medical thinking of Europe at this time. When Dr. Elisha Dick suggested a tracheotomy for his well-known patient, George Washington, Drs. James Craig and Gustavus Brown did not concur, instead treating him with blood-letting to release "evil humors" [20]. On December 14, 1799, the first President of the United States died of an acute upper airway obstruction secondary to a peritonsillar abscess [7]. His worsening symptoms happened within 36 hours of onset of sore throat and malaise, inability to speak, and difficulty breathing.

The terminology used to describe the procedure changed over time as well. Up until this time, the operation was known as a "Laryngotomy." In 1707, Pierre Dionis wrote that it was wrong to use this term and it should be called "bronchotomy" [6]. In 1718, Lorenz Heister wrote in the prestigious *Chirurgie* that the operation should be called tracheotomy and all other names should be discarded [21,22]. It was not until the nineteenth century that this term became accepted.

The British surgeon, George Martin, introduced the double lumen cannula with the advantage of an inner cannula that could be removed and cleaned, thus preventing tube obstruction with mucus [9]. A tube with a flange allowed easy placement of tapes to keep the tube in place and another one with a loose flange allowed some flexibility with neck movement. This important advance in postoperative care was quickly discarded and forgotten [7].

The period of dramatization (AD 1833–1932)

During the third stage of tracheotomy, it was an operation of life or death, performed only in emergencies on acutely obstructed airways. McKenzie summarized the general feelings of those times, writing, "the question always arises in the mind of the young surgeon whether the symptoms are sufficiently urgent to render the operation necessary" [9]. Having performed more than two hundred tracheotomies, Trousseau reported happily that one-fourth were successful [23]. In 1837, Curling discussed the respiratory distress associated with tetanus, including laryngospasm and dysfunctional accessory respiratory muscles. Although the description of symptoms favored the use of tracheotomy as a symptomatic treatment, the procedure was never carried out [24]. Brodie carried out tracheotomy in 1843 to successfully remove a swallowed 20 mm coin that had been lodged in a patient [25]. In 1869, Dr. Erichsen described four complications of tracheotomy: exposing the air tube, hemorrhage, opening of air passage, and placing the tracheotomy tube. He further recommended that the tube be cleaned with a sponge and solution of silver nitrate [26]. In 1888, Prince Frederick of Germany had a tracheotomy for a malignant laryngeal lesion. His treatment was more palliative than curative, and he did not live past 4 months; however, this foreshadowed palliative use of this procedure that is still prevalent today.

Over time, tracheotomy became an accepted technique to bypass upper airway obstruction caused by infection or foreign bodies, and to rest the larynx in chronic tuberculosis or

T. II. 449.

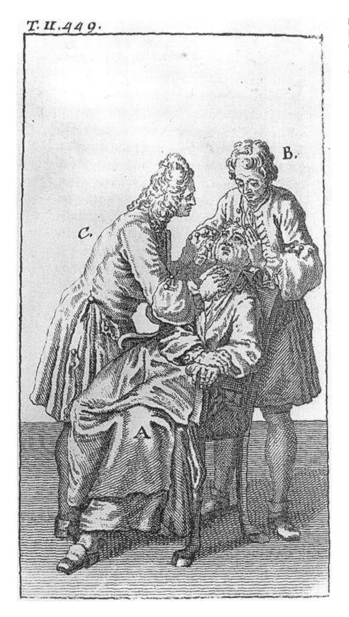

Figure 2 Performing a bronchotomy (tracheotomy). *Chirurgie Scènes de la vie médicale: Traité des opérations de chirurgie Paris*: G. Cavelier, 1731.

syphilis. Vehement arguments ensued in the literature over indications and technique. In 1860, the New Sydenham Society published over 38 papers devoted to discussing various techniques and indications for tracheotomy. The operative technique of tracheotomy was studied, refined, and described by Chevalier Jackson in 1909 [27]. Jackson defined factors that predisposed to complications, such as a high incision, using an improper cannula, poor postoperative care, and splitting of the cricoid cartilage. He designed a metal double lumen tube of proper length and curvature with just the right fitting to avoid excessive pressure on the anterior or posterior wall of the trachea and reduce the risk of ulceration and tracheal

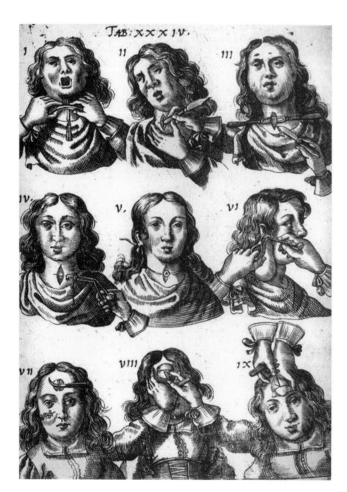

Figure 3 Ancient engraving illustrating a tracheotomy procedure. From *Armamentarium chirurgicum bipartitum*, 1666.

erosion. Jackson also developed a "J" tube with a long shaft that could bypass mid or lower tracheal obstruction, and he favored a vertical incision from the thyroid notch to the suprasternal notch for best visibility of the surgical field [27]. Jackson's teachings significantly reduced the complication rate and mortality rate of tracheotomy.

During the American Civil War from 1861 to 1865, tracheotomy was used by Union Army physicians to relieve respiratory distress in gunshot wounds of the head and neck. Despite improvements in technique, however, the First World War witnessed hesitation and even opposition to tracheotomy in war wound management.

Early in the twentieth century, diphtheria became controlled by immunization, while the discovery of sulfonamides helped curb other upper respiratory infections. The need for emergency tracheotomy became less common. For a brief period, tracheotomy was the only means of securing airways through general anesthesia, but the increasing popularity of endotracheal intubation replaced the need for tracheotomy. "The period of dramatization" was ending, although new antibiotics provided better prevention and control of infection in tracheotomy cases where the procedure was inevitable.

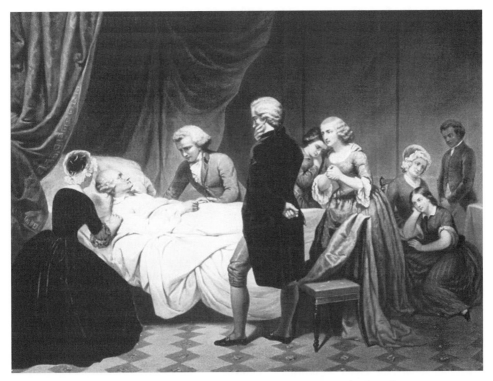

Figure 4 George Washington on his death bed: diagnosed with quinsy (peritonsilar abscess).

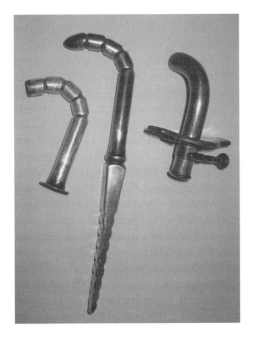

Figure 5 Durham Flexible Pilot (introducer) Lobster tail Tracheotomy tube, inner canula and introducer (circa 1890s). Photo Courtesy of Mr. Cedric Russell.

The period of enthusiasm (AD 1932–1965)

During the fourth stage in the history of tracheotomy the saying, "If you think tracheotomy … do it!" became popular. During this period, indications for tracheotomy were actively sought and the surgical and medical world became strong advocates for it. This period began in 1932 during the outbreak of bulbar poliomyelitis. Wilson suggested the use of tracheotomy to *prevent* impending pulmonary infection in poliomyelitis, as patients affected are unable to cough and raise secretions. He suggested that tracheotomy would provide an adequate airway and the patient could be managed by intermittent negative pressure respiration if provided with a cuffed tracheotomy tube and placed in an "iron lung." Thus, for the first time, tracheotomy was considered as an elective procedure [28]. Polio remained an epidemic until the early 1950s when the invention of positive pressure respiration together with tracheotomy greatly reduced mortality [29]. However, like diphtheria in previous years, the rate of poliomyelitis decreased to almost nil with the onset of universal vaccination.

Tracheotomy was openly advocated for tetanus, head, chest, and maxillofacial injuries, drug overdose, and following major surgery where airway patency was compromised [7]. During the Spanish Civil War in 1936–1939, the rules of triage for soldiers with maxillofacial injuries were modified. While they were waiting for surgery, the soldiers had high rates of aspiration and frequently suffered from respiratory distress. The use of tracheotomy decreased mortality rates for soldiers waiting for such surgeries [30]. This approach continued through the Second World War, where tracheotomy became an integral part of the management of soldiers with chest injury, burns, blast injuries, and traumatic wounds that caused retained pulmonary secretions to obstruct upper airways [31]. In 1943, Thomas C. Galloway recommended the use of tracheotomy for removal of bronchial secretions in myasthenia gravis and tetanus [29]. Carte and Guiseppi recognized the physiological benefits of tracheotomy, namely the reduction in dead space ventilation. This understanding led to the use of tracheotomy for chronic obstructive lung disease and severe pneumonia [32]. Tracheotomy became more prevalent as intensive care and post-anesthetic care units were established in the 1950s, with better care for tracheotomy patients [33].

The indications for tracheotomy were changing. Many infectious diseases that had previously caused upper airway obstruction were now controlled. As late as 1961, Meade, in a series of 212 cases showed that 41% of tracheotomies were still carried out on patients with upper airway obstruction due to tumor, infectious disease, and trauma, and 55% were performed to assist in mechanical ventilation [34].

The period of rationalization (AD 1965 to the present)

In 1965, it became apparent that oral or nasal endotracheal intubation was quicker and safer than tracheotomy, with a lower complication rate. So began the "period of rationalization," during which the merits of tracheotomy versus intubation have been debated. Improvements in tracheotomy tubes (e.g., the double lumen tube), improvement in cleaning and suction techniques, and use of biocompatible materials contributed significantly to the safety of the procedure. High-volume, low-pressure cuffs decreased the incidence of tracheal injury that can lead to scarring and stenosis by ensuring a stable airway seal without compromising perfusion pressure [35]. The flexible fiberoptic endoscope allowed atraumatic oral or nasal intubation in situations, such as cervical spine injuries, which previously necessitated tracheotomy.

Acute obstruction with impending asphyxia is no longer an indication for tracheotomy because alternatives, such as endotracheal intubation or cricothyroidotomy, are available. In fact, the emergency tracheotomy has become rare indeed. In a recent study of 1130 tracheotomies, Goldenberg *et al.* showed that 76% of tracheotomies were prophylactically performed on patients requiring prolonged mechanical ventilation while only 6% of patients were tracheotomized due to upper airway obstruction. Only 0.26% were performed on an emergency basis [36].

Percutaneous dilational tracheotomy (PDT) is an alternative to open tracheotomy because it can be comfortably performed at the bedside. In 1953, Seldinger introduced the technique of percutaneous guidewire needle placement for arterial catheterization [37]. Soon after, the guidewire technique (known as the "Seldinger technique") was adapted to percutaneous tracheotomy. The first modern PDT was reported by Shelden *et al.* in 1955, but the complication rate was very high due to perforation of the trachea and lacerations of adjacent structures [38]. In 1969, Toy and Weinstein developed a tapered straight dilator for performing percutaneous tracheotomy over a guiding catheter [39].

The technique of PDT using serial dilators over a guidewire was first described in 1985 by Ciaglia *et al.* [40]. In 1989, Schachner *et al.* developed a dilating tracheotomy forceps over a guidewire [41]. Studies of this new technique concluded that it was safe in elective circumstances, various medical personnel are able to carry out this procedure at the patient's bedside, there is reduced risk of infection, and the intercartilaginous membrane of the trachea heals well [42].

In 1990, Griggs *et al.* developed another guidewire dilating forceps for percutaneous tracheotomy [43]. The simplicity of this technique made tracheotomy more flexible and less traumatic. This technique is recommended and remains worthwhile in intensive care units [44,45]. As evolving medical literature debates the details, PDT is rapidly gaining acceptance as an alternative to the open tracheotomy in the treatment of patients requiring prolonged mechanical ventilation.

Conclusions

For more than 5000 years, tracheotomy has undergone changes in indications and techniques much like evolution in the practice of medicine itself. It could have potentially saved the life of the first American President if Dr. Elisha Dick had not faced opposition from his more senior colleagues. At times, dreaded, scorned, and carried out with extreme hesitancy, and in other instances, a noble and dramatic life-saving procedure, tracheotomy remains one of the most important and commonly performed surgical procedures to this day. It is a procedure carried out routinely in the operating room, intensive and intermediate care units, and in locations with minimal medical support during acute emergencies.

References

1. Pahor AL. Ear, nose and throat in Ancient Egypt. *J Laryngol Otol* 1992; **106**: 773–9.

2. McClelland RMA. *Progress in Anesthesiology Proceedings of the 4th World Congress of Anesthesiologists*. Amsterdam: Exerpta Medica, 1970; 105–96.

3. Wright J. *A History of Laryngology and Rhinology*. Philadelphia: Lea & Feiber, 1914; 65.

4. Gordon BL. *The Romance of Medicine*. Philadelphia: FA Davis, 1947; 461.

5. Galen. Introductio Seu Medicus. CG Kuhn (Trans) Leipzig, 1856, 406, Areataeus: *The*

Therapeutics of Acute Diseases. F Adam (Trans) London, The Syndenham Society, 1856; 406.

6. Stock CR. What is past is prologue: a short history of the development of tracheotomy. *Ear Nose Throat J* 1987; **66**(4): 166–9.

7. Frost EA. Tracing the tracheotomy. *Ann Otol Rhinol Laryngol* 1976; **85**(5 Pt.1): 618–24.

8. Aurelianus C. *De Morb. Acut* (Circa 5th Century AD) Book 53, chapter 4.

9. McKenzie M. *Diseases of the Pharynx, Larynx and Trachea.* New York: Wood and Co., 1880; 397.

10. Bradby M. History of tracheotomy. *Nurs Times* 1966; **62**: 1548–50.

11. Goodall EW. The story of tracheotomy. *Br J Child Dis* 1934; **31**: 167–76, 253–72.

12. Linhart W. *Compendium der Chirurg. Operation Lehre.* Vienna, 1877.

13. Stevenson RS, Guthrie D. *History of Otolaryngology.* Edinburgh: E & S Livingston, 1949; 1731.

14. Pierson DJ. Tracheotomy from A to Z: historical context and current challenges. *Respir Care* 2005; **50**: 473–5.

15. Habicott N. *Sur la bronchotomie, Vulgairment Dicte Larynotomie,* ou Perforation De Flute Au Tayau Du Pulman, Paris 1620.

16. Bonetus T. Sepulchetum Sive Anatomica Practica t.i. lib. *2 De Respiratione Laesa,* Obs. I, Geneva, 1700; 483.

17. Borman J, Davidson JT. A history of tracheotomy: Si Spiritum Ducit Vivit. *Br J Anesthesiol* 1963; **35**: 388–90.

18. Home F. *An Inquiry into the Natural Causes and Cure of Croup.* Edinburgh: Kincaid and Bell, 1765.

19. Wendt A. *Historia Tracheotomiae nuperrime Administratae,* in 8 vo. Vrasislaviae, 1774.

20. Jafek BW. Minutiae in otolaryngology. In: Jafek BW, Stark A, eds. *ENT Secrets.* Philadelphia: Hanley & Belfus, 1996: 425–30.

21. Dionis P. *Cours d'operatione de chirurgiris,* ed. Paris: L dHoury, 1751.

22. Heister L. *General System of Surgery,* Vol. 2, 8th edn. London: Printed for W Innys, J Richardson, C Davis, and J Clark, 1768; 52.

23. Trousseau A. *Lectures on Clinical Medicine,* Vol. 2. JR Cormack (trans). London: The New Syndenham Society, 1869, 598.

24. Curling TB. *A Treatise on Tetanus.* Philadelphia, PA: Haswell, Barrington & Haswell, 1837.

25. Conacher ID. Brodie's tracheotomy. *J R Soc Med* 1992; **85**: 570–2.

26. Erichsen JE. *The Science and Art of Surgery.* Philadelphia: Henry C Lea, 1869; 919.

27. Jackson C. Tracheotomy. *Laryngoscope* 1909; **19**: 285.

28. Wilson JL. Acute anterior poliomyelitis treatment of bulbar and high spinal types. *N Engl J Med* 1932; **206**: 887.

29. Galloway TC. Tracheotomy in bulbar poliomyelitis. *JAMA* 1943; **128**: 1096–7.

30. Booth JB. Tracheotomy and tracheal intubation in military history. *J R Soc Med* 2000; **93**: 380–3.

31. Pratt LW. Tracheotomy: historical review. *Am Laryngol* 2008; **118**: 1597–606.

32. Carte BN, Guiseppi J. Tracheotomy, a useful procedure in thoracic surgery with particular reference to its employment in crushing injuries of the thorax. *J Thorac Surg* 1951; **21**: 495.

33. Collins CG. Rationale and value of tracheotomy in severe preeclampsia and eclampsia. *Postgrad Med* 1955; **17**: 259–66.

34. Meade JW. Tracheotomy – Its complications and their management. *N Engl J Med* 1961; **265**: 519–23.

35. Heffner JE, Miller KS, Sahn SA. Tracheotomy in the intensive care unit: complications. *Chest* 1986; **90**: 430–6.

36. Goldenberg D, Ari EG, Golz A, Danino J, Netzer A, Joachims HZ. Tracheotomy complications: a retrospective study of 1130 cases. *Otolaryngol Head Neck Surg* 2000; **123**: 495–500.

37. Seldinger SI. Catheter replacement of the needle in percutaneous arteriography. *Acta Radiol* 1953; **39**: 368–76.

38. Shelden CH, Pudenz RH, Freshwater DB, *et al*. New method for tracheotomy. *J Neurosurg* 1955; **12**: 428–31.

39. Toy FJ, Weinstein JD. A percutaneous tracheotomy device. *Surgery* 1969; **65**: 384–9.

40. Ciaglia P, Firshing R, Syniec C. Elective percutaneous dilational tracheotomy: a new simple bedside procedure. *Chest* 1985; **87**: 715–19.

41. Schachner A, Ovil Y, Sidi J, *et al*. Percutaneous tracheotomy: a new method. *Crit Care Med* 1989; **17**: 1052–6.

42. Kost KM. Endoscopic percutaneous dilational tracheotomy: a perspective evaluation of 500 consecutive cases. *Laryngoscope* 2005; **115**: 1–20.

43. Griggs WM, Worthley LIG, Gilligan JE, *et al*. A simple percutaneous tracheotomy technique. *Surg Gynecol Obstet* 1990; **170**: 543–5.

44. Van Heerbeek N, Fikkers GB, Van Den Hoogen JA, *et al*. The guide wire dilating forceps technique of percutaneous tracheotomy. *Am J Surg* 1999; **277**: 311–15.

45. Kumar M, Jaffery A, Jones M. Short-term complications of percutaneous tracheotomy: experience of a district general hospital-otolaryngology department. *J Laryngol Otol* 2002; **116**: 1025–7.

Anatomy of the anterior and lateral neck

Elliot Regenbogen

Case presentation

A 47-year-old female inpatient with a history of liver transplantation secondary to hemo-chromatosis, hypertension, insulin-dependent diabetes mellitus, and chronic renal insuffi-ciency, developed hemoptysis and brisk hemorrhage from her tracheotomy site. Initially, the patient was admitted to the hospital with pneumonia-induced pulmonary failure that necessitated endotracheal intubation. Owing to the prolonged need for ventilatory support, a tracheotomy was performed 34 days before the onset of hemorrhage. An extra-long cuffed tracheotomy tube was placed between the third and fourth tracheal cartilages. The patient's hospital course was complicated by acute chronic renal failure that required initiation of hemodialysis, severe fluid overload, congestive heart failure, and adult respiratory distress syndrome (ARDS). At the time of consultation, she was bleeding overtly from her trache-otomy site.

The skin and superficial fascia of the neck

Skin incisions for tracheotomy may be placed vertically in the midline or horizontally in the direction of skin tension lines (Langer's lines). The next layer divided is the fatty subcutaneous tissue, which can vary in thickness. The platysma muscle embedded deep within this layer can also be of varied thickness but is usually very thin or absent in the midline. This muscle begins over the clavicles and inserts over the mandible. The platysma muscle together with the subcutaneous tissue comprises the superficial fascia of the head and neck.

The deep fascia and spaces below the hyoid bone

The deep fascia forms more distinct layers: superficial, pretracheal/middle, prevertebral/deep, and carotid sheaths [1].

The superficial and prevertebral layers of the deep fascia originate from the vertebral spinous processes and ligamentum nuchae and completely encircle the neck.

The superficial layer splits to surround the sternocleidomastoid and strap/infrahyoid muscles. The portion anterior to these muscles attaches superiorly to the hyoid bone and inferiorly to the sternum. The portion overlying the posterior surface of the strap muscles

Tracheotomy Management: A Multidisciplinary Approach, ed. Peggy A. Seidman, David Goldenberg and Elizabeth H. Sinz. Published by Cambridge University Press.

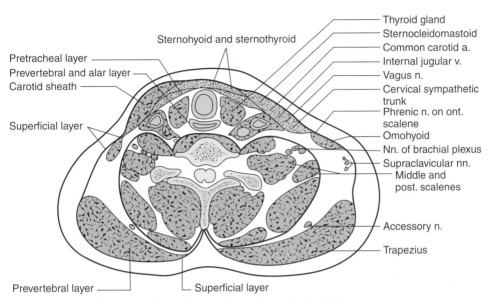

Figure 1.1 Cervical fascia below the hyoid bone, adapted from Hollinshead [1].

(i.e., pretracheal layer) ends inferiorly in the superior mediastinum and superiorly upon the thyroid cartilage and hyoid bone.

The posterior portion of the superficial fascia splits to surround the jugular vein, common carotid artery, and vagus nerve to form the anterior and posterior lateral walls of the carotid sheath. A bridge between these two walls forms the medial wall of the carotid sheath.

The prevertebral layer of fascia turns medially behind the carotid sheath separated from it by loose connective tissue.

Spaces and compartments

Visceral compartment

Above the level of the inferior thyroid arteries, the area of loose connective tissue surrounding the thyroid gland, trachea, and esophagus is known as the visceral compartment.

Below this level, the compartment is divided into two portions separated by dense connective tissue, which attaches the esophageal wall laterally to the prevertebral layer of fascia. The anterior part of the compartment surrounds the trachea and anterior wall of the esophagus; this is known as the pretracheal space. The retropharyngeal/retroesophageal or collectively the retrovisceral space is the posterior part of the compartment, behind the lower part of the pharynx and esophagus.

Pretracheal and retrovisceral spaces

The superior limit of the pretracheal space is the attachment of the strap muscles and their fascia to the thyroid cartilage and hyoid bone. The inferior limit is the anterior portion of the superior mediastinum.

From the skull base the posterior portion of the visceral compartment in the neck extends inferiorly behind the pharynx, the retropharyngeal space, and continues as the retroesophageal space. Both the pretracheal and retrovisceral spaces descend into the superior mediastinum acting as important potential conduits of head and neck infections.

Infrahyoid, "strap," muscles

The muscles deep to the platysma, which lie centrally in the neck overlying the larynx, thyroid gland, and trachea, are known as the infrahyoid or "strap" muscles.

The four muscles in this group are the sternohyoid, sternothyroid, thyrohyoid, and omohyoid.

The sternohyoid originates on the posterior sternum and medial end of the clavicle and inserts on the hyoid bone. The omohyoid muscle is deep to this, at first parallel with its superior belly and then laterally as it continues as its inferior belly.

The sternothyroid and thyrohyoid muscles are deep to the sternohyoid and the superior belly of the omohyoid muscles. The sternothyroid arises from the posterior surface of the sternum below the origin of the sternohyoid and inserts on the oblique line of the thyroid cartilage; the thyrohyoid arises from the oblique line and continues upward to an insertion upon the hyoid bone.

Arteries and veins

Subclavian artery and branches

The right subclavian artery is a continuation of the brachiocephalic (innominate) trunk behind the sternoclavicular articulation; it arches upward and laterally, leaving the neck by

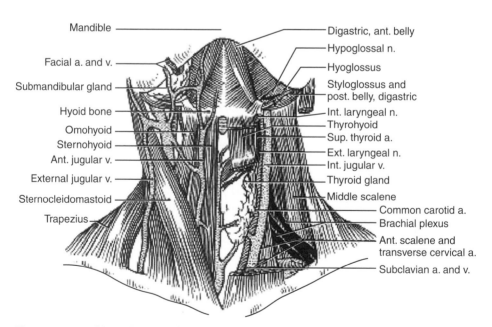

Figure 1.2 View of the neck, adapted from Hollinshead [1].

crossing the first rib, becoming the axillary. The left subclavian artery comes directly off the aortic arch, arising lower than the right one, traversing the mediastinum eventually crossing the first rib to become the axillary.

Tracheoinnominate artery erosion

Erosion of a tracheotomy tube through the tracheal wall and into the innominate artery is one of the most feared late complications. The risk of tracheoinnominate artery erosion is increased by low placement, excessive movement, or an overinflated tracheotomy tube cuff. The artery crosses the trachea at about the ninth tracheal ring. This complication occurs in less than 1% of all patients undergoing tracheotomy. The vast majority of cases (approximately 75%) will occur within 3–4 weeks of tracheotomy placement. The mortality rate approaches 100%, even when surgical intervention is undertaken [2].

Vertebral artery

The vertebral artery is typically the first branch to arise from the posterior part of the first portion of the subclavian. It runs upward to enter the foramen of a transverse process – anywhere from the seventh to the fourth.

Thyrocervical trunk

The most common origin of the thyrocervical trunk is the upper and anterior portion of the first portion of the subclavian artery. It divides into several branches, with great variation. The arterial branches are the suprascapular (transverse scapular), transverse cervical, and inferior thyroid. The suprascapular and transverse cervical branches may arise individually or as one trunk either from the thyrocervical trunk or directly from the subclavian artery.

Inferior thyroid artery

The inferior thyroid artery branch of the thyrocervical trunk runs upward in the neck in front of the vertebral artery. It gives off an ascending cervical branch and then passes medially and downward to make an arch behind the carotid sheath, penetrating the prevertebral fascia,

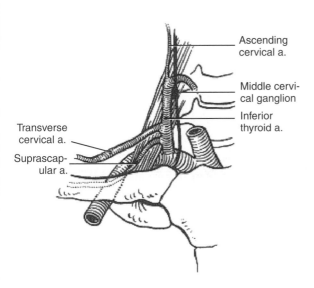

Ascending cervical a.

Middle cervical ganglion

Inferior thyroid a.

Transverse cervical a.

Suprascapular a.

Figure 1.3 The thyrocervical trunk, adapted from Hollinshead [2].

and reaching the posterior aspect of the thyroid gland where it further divides in an intimate but sometimes variable relationship with the recurrent laryngeal nerve.

Suprascapular and transverse cervical artery

The suprascapular (transverse scapular) artery branch of the thyrocervical trunk, passes across the neck in front of the brachial plexus and third part of the subclavian artery and downward behind the clavicle to reach the muscles of the scapula.

The transverse cervical artery runs almost transversely across the neck somewhat higher and above the level of the upper border of the clavicle. It passes across the posterior triangle of the neck to reach the deep surface of the trapezius muscle.

Arteries of the central neck

Common carotid artery

The right common carotid artery arises from the brachiocephalic (innominate) artery behind the sternoclavicular joint while the left arises directly from the arch of the aorta.

At the base of the neck, the two common carotid arteries are covered by fascia, the sternocleidomastoid and strap muscles. The artery bifurcates at the level of the hyoid bone into external and internal branches; at this point is only covered by skin, fascia, and platysma.

Each common carotid artery is enclosed in a carotid sheath. Within separate compartments of the carotid sheath are the internal jugular vein laterally and the vagus nerve behind and somewhat between the two. Anteriomedially the common carotid artery is related to the trachea, thyroid gland, and larynx.

Carotid bifurcation

The common carotid artery gives off two branches, the internal and external carotids. The bifurcation of the common carotid artery usually occurs at about the level of the hyoid bone. The carotid body is on the posteromedial surface of the common carotid artery at its bifurcation and contains chemosensory receptors, which respond to hypoxia. The carotid sinus is part of the carotid artery and responds to pressure, reducing blood pressure.

Internal carotid artery

Ascending from the carotid bifurcation the internal carotid artery is laterally crossed by the hypoglossal nerve, occipital artery, and posterior belly of the digastric muscle, stylohyoid muscle, and posterior auricular artery. At the skull base, the external carotid artery is separated from the internal carotid artery by the stylopharyngeus muscle, associated glosso-pharyngeal nerve, pharyngeal branch of the vagus, and stylohyoid ligament.

External carotid artery and branches

Ascending from the carotid bifurcation the external carotid passes anteriomedial to the internal carotid, deep to the posterior belly of the digastric muscle and stylohyoid muscle. It then crosses the styloglossus and stylopharyngeus muscles on their lateral surface, which separates the internal and external carotid, and then parallels the ramus of the mandible passing into the deeper portion of the parotid gland.

Branches of the external carotid artery in ascending order include the superior thyroid, ascending pharyngeal, lingual, facial, occipital, posterior auricular, superficial temporal and maxillary.

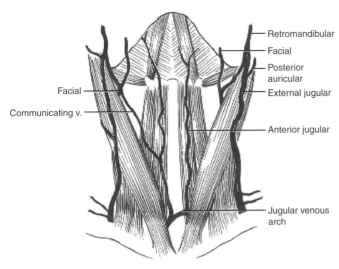

Figure 1.4 Superficial veins of the neck, adapted from Hollinshead [1].

Superficial veins of the central neck

External jugular vein

A merger of contributions from the retromandibular (posterior facial), posterior auricular, facial, maxillary, and internal jugular veins form the external jugular vein. The external jugular vein usually terminates in the subclavian vein or the internal jugular vein.

Anterior jugular vein

Venous contributions forming the anterior jugular veins include superficial veins of the suprahyoid region, the retromandibular, facial, or parotid veins. The anterior jugular veins descend parallel to each other on the infrahyoid muscles or more laterally on the anterior borders of the sternocleidomastoid muscles. Lower in the neck the two converge and usually unite by a transverse jugular arch, which can be encountered in a low tracheotomy. Below this, the anterior jugular empties into the subclavian vein between the internal and external jugular veins. These veins are often encountered when performing a tracheotomy.

Deep veins of the central neck

Internal jugular vein

As they emerge from the anterior portion of the jugular foramen in the skull base the ninth, tenth, and eleventh cranial nerves separate the internal jugular vein from the internal carotid artery. Lower down in the neck the internal jugular veins are lateral to the internal carotid and common carotid arteries.

As the jugular vein assumes a position lateral to the artery, the vagus nerve lies behind and somewhat between the two vessels, just as it does lower down in the neck in relation to this vein and the common carotid artery.

At about the level of the hyoid bone the internal jugular vein receives the facial vein, superior thyroid vein, and often pharyngeal and lingual veins.

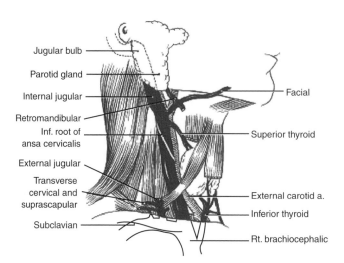

Figure 1.5 Deeper veins of the neck, adapted from Hollinshead [1].

Jugular bulb

Parotid gland

Internal jugular

Retromandibular

Inf. root of ansa cervicalis

External jugular

Transverse cervical and suprascapular

Subclavian

Facial

Superior thyroid

External carotid a.

Inferior thyroid

Rt. brachiocephalic

Nerves of the central neck

Cutaneous innervation

Sensory contributions of the second and third cervical nerve to the transverse cervical branch of the cervical plexus provide cutaneous innervation of the neck.

Tenth nerve and its branches

Tracing the vagus nerve as it exits the skull base via the jugular foramen, the nerve enlarges to form the inferior or nodose ganglion. Here, the vagus is medial to the internal carotid artery and internal jugular vein and between the glossopharyngeal and accessory nerves. As it descends, the vagus will be positioned between the carotid artery and jugular vein.

The inferior ganglion of the vagus gives off the superior laryngeal nerve branch. The superior laryngeal nerve descends initially behind the internal carotid artery eventually dividing into external (motor) and internal (sensory) branches. The external branch further descends with the superior thyroid artery giving off branches to the inferior pharyngeal constrictor muscle and cricothyroid muscles. The internal branch is sensory to the supraglottic mucosa entering the larynx via the thyrohyoid membrane with the superior laryngeal artery.

Lower in the neck the vagus nerve gives off the recurrent laryngeal nerve branch, which has a different course on each side of the neck. On the right, it leaves the vagus in the neck in front of the subclavian artery and loops below and behind the artery to ascend obliquely to the posterolateral aspect of the trachea and pass upward toward the larynx. The left recurrent nerve arises in the mediastinum from the left vagus as it passes across the arch of the aorta and then runs upward alongside the trachea to reach the larynx.

Twelfth nerve and the ansa cervicalis

The hypoglossal nerve emerges from the skull base through the hypoglossal canal medial to the internal jugular vein and internal carotid artery. Close to the canal, it receives branches from upper cervical nerves, which then leave it as the superior root of the ansa cervicalis, the nerve to the thyrohyoid and the nerve to the geniohyoid. The hypoglossal nerve itself supplies motor function to the tongue muscles. A branch from the superior root of the ansa cervicalis supplies the upper belly of the omohyoid muscle and upper portions of the sternohyoid and sternothyroid, while other branches from the ansa cervicalis supply the inferior belly of the omohyoid and lower portions of the sternohyoid and sternothyroid. As both roots of the ansa are composed of cervical nerve fibers, infrahyoid muscles are innervated entirely through cervical nerves and not by the hypoglossal nerve.

Visceral structures of the neck

Thyroid gland

The strap muscles of the neck, except the thyrohyoid muscle, cover the thyroid gland as it lies below and to the sides of the thyroid cartilage. The gland consists of a right and left lobe joined by the thyroid isthmus immediately below the cricoid cartilage, overlying the trachea. Pathologies of the thyroid gland can have a direct impact on exposure of the trachea during tracheotomy.

The blood supply to the thyroid gland is through the inferior thyroid artery, and superior thyroid artery (described above).

When present, the thyroid ima artery may be an accessory to the inferior thyroid artery or it may replace it. It usually arises from the innominate on the right side, ascending in front of the trachea. It is important to feel for this vessel during tracheotomy as it is present in 3% to 10% of the population.

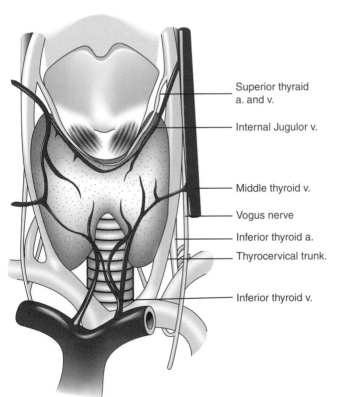

Figure 1.6 Arteries and veins of the thryoid gland, adapted from Hollinshead [1].

Superior thyraid a. and v.

Internal Jugulor v.

Middle thyroid v.

Vogus nerve

Inferior thyroid a.

Thyrocervical trunk.

Inferior thyroid v.

The venous drainage of the thyroid consists of the superior, middle, and inferior thyroid veins. The two inferior thyroid veins usually remain independent but freely anastomose with each other forming the plexus thyroideus impar in front of the trachea. This can be a significant source of bleeding during tracheotomy.

The larynx

Thyroid cartilage

The thyroid cartilage forms most of the anterior and lateral walls of the larynx. The thyrohyoid membrane located in the space between the thyroid cartilage and hyoid bone just above, is attached between the two.

In young children, the hyoid bone is much closer and may overlap the thyroid cartilage, making the thyroid cartilage the least palpable structure instead of the most prominent as it usually is in older children and adults.

Structures within the boundaries of the thyroid cartilage include the epiglottis, false vocal folds, ventricles, true vocal folds, arytenoid, corniculate, and cuneiform cartilages.

Cricoid cartilage

Unlike the thyroid cartilage, the cricoid is a complete ring. The shape of the cricoid cartilage is described as that of a signet ring, narrow in the front and tall posteriorly. Posterolaterally the cricoid ring articulates with the inferior horn of the thyroid cartilage at the cricothyroid articulation. Anterior to the articulation, the only attachment is the cricothyroid membrane (ligament).

The cricoid cartilage is the narrowest part of the trachea with an average adult diameter of 17 mm in men and 13 mm in women [4].

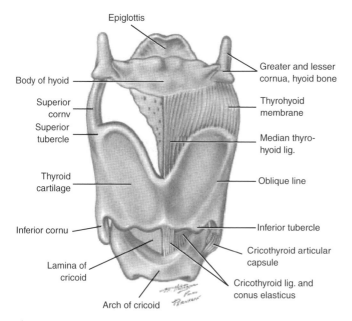

Figure 1.7 Cartilages and ligaments of the larynx, adapted from Hollinshead [1].

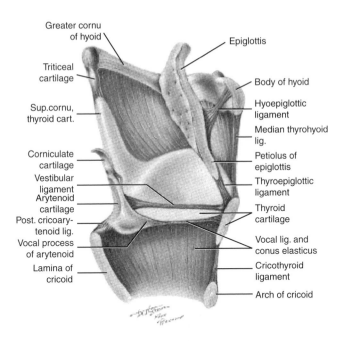

Figure 1.8 Cartilages and ligaments of the larynx in sagittal section, adapted from Hollinshead [1].

Labels on figure:
Greater cornu of hyoid
Triticeal cartilage
Sup.cornu, thyroid cart.
Corniculate cartilage
Vestibular ligament
Arytenoid cartilage
Post. cricoary-tenoid lig.
Vocal process of arytenoid
Lamina of cricoid
Epiglottis
Body of hyoid
Hyoepiglottic ligament
Median thyrohyoid lig.
Petiolus of epiglottis
Thyroepiglottic ligament
Thyroid cartilage
Vocal lig. and conus elasticus
Cricothyroid ligament
Arch of cricoid

Posteriorly, the cricothyroid membrane is overlapped externally by the cricothyroid muscle, which also connects these two cartilages. Anterolaterally, the cricothyroid membrane is subcutaneous. Cricothyroidotomy, an emergency surgical airway procedure, is performed through this membrane.

Trachea and esophagus

Tracheal histology, innervation, and vascular supply

Pseudostratified ciliated columnar epithelium lines the trachea. Secretory cells to produce mucus, and ciliated cells, to propel trapped foreign bodies towards the pharynx, constitute the bulk of the epithelium. Fibroelastic lamina propria and submucosa, which contains cartilage and muscle, compose the subepithelial tissue [6].

The vagus and recurrent laryngeal nerves innervate the trachea. Sympathetic trunks supply sympathetic nerves and vagal branches provide parasympathetic fibers. Sympathetic nerve activity relaxes tracheal smooth muscle; parasympathetic nerve activity contracts it [3].

Tracheal branches of the inferior thyroid and bronchial arteries supply the trachea. Inferior thyroid veins drain the trachea and can unite into a plexus thyroideus impar anterior to the trachea. The trachea is richly endowed with lymphatics, which empty into pretracheal or paratracheal lymph nodes [3].

Gross anatomy

The trachea begins at the lower border of the cricoid cartilage. The trachea is made up of 16–22 C-shaped rings of cartilage anteriorly joined by the annular ligaments and posteriorly by the trachealis muscle. Proximally, the trachea is close to the skin and as it descends it angles to a near midcoronal level at the carina.

The trachea is located in the midline position, but often can be deviated to the right at the level of the aortic arch, with a greater degree of displacement in the setting of an atherosclerotic aorta, advanced age or in the presence of severe chronic obstructive pulmonary disease.

As a continuation of the pharynx, the esophagus begins below the lower border of the cricoid cartilage behind the trachea and, unlike the trachea, does not run down the midline of the neck but curves slightly to the left.

A tracheoesophageal fistula is a relatively rare complication in which development of a connection between the trachea and esophagus occurs. Injury to the posterior tracheal wall may occur due to tracheotomy, from excessive cuff pressure or positioning of the tip of the tracheotomy tube against the posterior tracheal wall.

In the average adult, the distance from cricoid to carina is approximately 11 cm, with a range of 10–13 cm. On average, the trachea is 2.3 cm wide and 1.8 cm from posterior membrane to the anterior cartilaginous aspect. The trachea is wider in men than in women [6,7].

Anterior to the trachea in the neck is the isthmus of the thyroid gland at about the level of the second to fourth tracheal cartilages; below this the inferior thyroid veins, lymph nodes, and sometimes a thyroid ima artery. Anterior to all of these are the strap muscles.

Lateral to the trachea in the neck are the lobes of the thyroid gland, great vessels, and recurrent laryngeal nerves (see Figure 1.6).

The innominate artery crosses the trachea either behind the sternum or in the lower portion of the neck. During tracheotomy the careful surgeon will palpate this region to assess the presence of a high riding innominate artery. The jugular venous arch connecting the two anterior jugular veins lies superficial to the strap muscles just above the suprasternal notch.

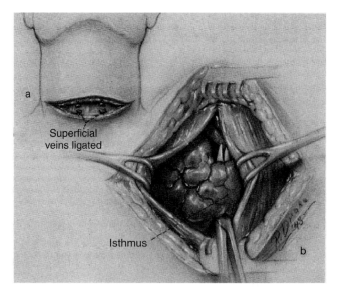

a

Superficial
veins ligated

Isthmus

b

Figure 1.9 Thyroid gland adapted from Hollinshead [1].

Neck anatomy and its relevance to tracheotomy

The basic anatomic relationships previously discussed need to be kept in mind in performing a tracheotomy (Figure 1.10). High tracheotomies, done much above the level of the thyroid isthmus, are generally felt to be associated with a higher rate of tracheal stenosis. Lower placement will encounter more vascular structures such as the thyroid veins, anterior jugular arch, or a high innominate artery. Horizontal skin incisions tend to be more cosmetic, although the external jugular veins and lateral anatomic structures must be considered during dissection. Vertical skin incisions tend to be avascular.

Surgical tracheotomy tubes are typically placed in the region of the second to fourth tracheal rings. This technique may entail removal of tracheal cartilage, division of tracheal cartilage, or creation of a cartilaginous flap. The thyroid isthmus may be divided or retracted. Percutaneous tracheotomy tubes are typically placed between the first and second or between the second and third tracheal cartilages utilizing progressive dilation of the space. A cricothyroidotomy places a smaller tube through the cricothyroid membrane [8].

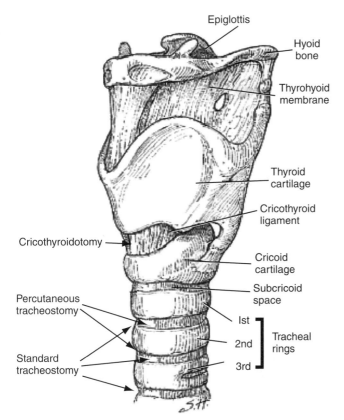

Epiglottis

Hyoid bone

Thyrohyoid membrane

Thyroid cartilage

Cricothyroid ligament

Cricothyroidotomy

Cricoid cartilage

Subcricoid space

Percutaneous tracheostomy

Standard tracheostomy

Ist

2nd

3rd

Tracheal rings

Figure 1.10 Cricothyroidotomy, adapted from Epstein [3].

Dimensions of the trachea

At birth, the inferior margin of the cricoid is at C4 and by adulthood at C6–7. At birth to 3 months, the length is 5.7 cm on average. Girls' tracheas stop growing at 14 years, whereas boys' stop elongating at this age but continue to enlarge. Tracheal length is strongly correlated to body height in children and adolescents [3].

Normal adult tracheal measurements are reviewed in Table 1.1 [9].

Table 1.1 Adult tracheal measurements

Normal adult tracheal measurements	
Length	
Total	8–13 cm
Extrathoracic	2–4 cm
Intrathoracic	6–9 cm
Diameter	
Men	
Average	19.5 mm
Coronal	13–25 mm
Sagittal	13–27 mm
Women	
Average	17.5 mm
Coronal	10–21 mm
Sagittal	10–23 mm
Adapted from reference [9].	

Tracheotomy tube selection

In infants and children, the diameter and length of the tracheotomy tube can be critical to the success of the procedure. Neonatal tracheotomy tubes are cuffless, have an outer diameter of 4.5–6.5 mm and a length of 30–36 mm. Pediatric size tracheotomy tubes have similar diameters at the smaller size but are longer in length. Cuffed pediatric tracheotomy tubes begin at an outer diameter of 5.9 mm. French sizing is three times the outer diameter.

For an adult, given the greater diameter of the trachea and availability of cuffed tracheotomy tubes, the diameter of the tracheotomy tube is less critical. Length may be more important for reasons such as obesity, presence of neck tumor, cervical kyphosis, tracheomalacia, tracheal stenosis, congenital anomaly, trauma, and infection.

Table 1.2 Approximate size of endotracheal and tracheotomy tubes for infants and children*

Age	Endotracheal¥	Shiley	Aberdeen	Hollinger
Premature	11–13	00		00
Newborn	14	0	3.5	0
Newborn–3 months	15–16	0	3.5	1
3–10 months	17	1	4.0	2
10–12 months	18	2	4.5	3
13–24 months	20	3	5.0	3
2–3 years	22	4	5.0	4
4–5 years	24	4	5.0	4
6–7 years	26	4	5.0	4
8–9 years	28	4	6.0	5
10–11 years	30	6	6.0	6
12 years and over	32	6	7.0	6

Adapted from reference [10].

*Based on outer diameter or circumference (French no.)
¥French no.

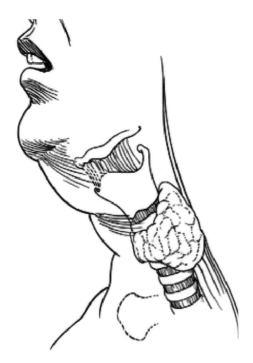

Figure 1.11 In the obese or a kyphotic neck, the distance from trachea to skin will be increased. In this case a cricoid hook can be used to pull the trachea anteriorly. Use of a longer tube is often necessary and fiberoptic bronchoscopy to confirm proper endoluminal placement is recommended. Adapted from Walts et al. [12].

Table 1.3

The left-hand margin groups the products as **PLASTIC** (Great Ormond Street through TracoeMini) and **SILVER** (Alder Hey through Sheffield).

Product	Measurement	Preterm-1 month	1-6 months	6-18 months	18 mths - 3 yrs	3-6 years	6-9 years	9-12 years	12-14 years
Trachea (Transverse Diameter mm)		5	5-6	6-7	7-8	8-9	9-10	10-13	13
Great Ormond Street	ID (mm)	3.0	3.5	4.0	4.5	5.0	5.5	6.0	7.0
	OD (mm)	4.5	5.0	6.0	6.7	7.5	8.0	8.7	10.7
Shiley	Size	3.0	3.5	4.0	4.5	5.0	5.5	6.0	6.5
	ID (mm)	3.0	3.5	4.0	4.5	5.0	5.5	6.0	6.5
	OD (mm)	4.5	5.2	5.9	6.5	7.1	7.7	8.3	9.0
	Length (mm) Neonatal	30	32	34	36				
*Cuffed Tube Available — Paediatric		39	40	41*	42*	44*	46*		
Long Paediatric						50*	52*	54*	56*
Portex (Blue Line)	ID (mm)	3.0	3.5	4.0	4.5	5.0	5.0	6.0	7.0
	OD (mm)	4.2	4.9	5.5	6.2	6.9	6.9	8.3	9.7
Portex (555)	Size	2.5	3.0	3.5	4.0	4.5	5.0	5.5	
	ID (mm)	2.5	3.0	3.5	4.0	4.5	5.0	5.5	
	OD (mm)	4.5	5.2	5.8	6.5	7.1	7.7	8.3	
	Length Neonatal	30	32	34	36				
	Paediatric	30	36	40	44	48	50	52	
Bivona	Size	2.5	3.0	3.5	4.0	4.5	5.0	5.5	
	ID (mm)	2.5	3.0	3.5	4.0	4.5	5.0	5.5	
	OD (mm)	4.0	4.7	5.3	6.0	6.7	7.3	8.0	
All sizes available with Fome Cuff, Aire Cuff & TTS Cuff — Length Neonatal		30	32	34	36				
	Paediatric	38	39	40	41	42	44	46	
Bivona Hyperflex	ID (mm)	2.5	3.0	3.5	4.0	4.5	5.0	5.5	
	Usable Length (mm)	55	60	65	70	75	80	85	
Bivona Flextend	ID (mm)	2.5	3.0	3.5	4.0	4.5	5.0	5.5	
	Shaft Length (mm)	38	39	40	41	42	44	46	
	Flextend Length (mm)	10	10	15	15	17.5	20	20	
TracoeMini	ID (mm)	2.5	3.0	3.5	4.0	4.5	5.0	5.5	6.0
	OD (mm)	3.6	4.3	5.0	5.6	6.3	7.0	7.6	8.4
	Length (mm) Neonatal (350)	30	32	34	36				
	Paediatric (355)	32	36	40	44	48	50	55	62
Alder Hey	FG		12-14	16	18	20	22	24	
Negus	FG		16	18	20	22	24	26	28
Chevalier Jackson	FG	14	16	18	20	22	24	26	28
Sheffield	FG		12-14	16	18	20	22	24	26
	ID (mm)		2.9-3.6	4.2	4.9	6.0	6.3	7.0	7.6
Cricoid (AP Diameter)	ID (mm)	3.6-4.8	4.8-5.8	5.8-6.5	6.5-7.4	7.4-8.2	8.2-9.0	9.0-10.7	10.7
Bronchoscope (Storz)	Size	2.5	3.0	3.5	4.0	4.5	5.0	6.0	6.0
	ID (mm)	3.5	4.3	5.0	6.0	6.6	7.1	7.5	7.5
	OD (mm)	4.2	5.0	5.7	6.7	7.3	7.8	8.2	8.2
Endotracheal Tube (Portex)	ID (mm)	2.5	3.0	3.5	4.0	4.5	5.0	6.0	7.0, 8.0
	OD (mm)	3.4	4.2	4.8	5.4	6.2	6.8	8.2	9.6, 10.8

Adapted from reference [11].

Conclusion

After temporary control of the hemorrhage was accomplished by tracheotomy cuff inflation, bedside fiberoptic bronchoscopy was performed and showed a distal tracheal blood clot but no active extravasation. Emergent angiography was significant for an innominate artery pseudoaneurysm adjacent to the tip of the endotracheal tube, a finding suggestive of tracheoinnominate fistula. Given the patient's overall frail medical condition and poor surgical risk for an open mediastinal operation, an endovascular approach was chosen for treatment [13]. A thorough knowledge of anatomy and anatomical variations of the head and neck is essential to avoid or assess complications arising from tracheotomies.

References

1   Hollinshead W. *Henry Anatomy: Anatomy for Surgeons*, Vol. 1, 3rd edn. Philadelphia: Harper and Row, 1982.

2   Sue RD, Susanto I. Long-term complications of artificial airways. *Clin Chest Med* 2003; **24**(3): 457–71.

3   Epstein SK. Anatomy and physiology of tracheostomy. *Respir Care* 2005; **50**(3): 476–82.

4   Campos JH. Update on tracheobronchial anatomy and flexible fiberoptic bronchoscopy in thoracic anesthesia. *Curr Opin Anaesthesiol* 2009; **22**: 4–10.

5   Michael HJ, Strollo D. Imaging of the normal trachea. *J Thorac Imaging* 1995; **10**: 171–9.

6   Rood S. Anatomy for tracheotomy. In: Myers E, Stool SE, Johnson JT, eds. *Tracheotomy*. New York: Churchill Livingstone, 1985; 89–97.

7   Streitz Jr JM, Shapshay SM. Airway injury after tracheotomy and endotracheal intubation. *Surg Clin North Am* 1991; **71**(6): 1211–30.

8   Johnson JT. Alternatives to tracheotomy: cricothyroidotomy. In: Myers E, Stool SE, Johnson JT, eds. *Tracheotomy*. New York: Churchill Livingstone, 1985; 83–8.

9   Boiselle PM. Imaging of the large airways. *Clin Chest Med* 2008; **29**: 181–93.

10 Bluestone CD, Stool SE, Scheetz MD. *Pediatric Otolaryngology*. Pennsylvania: WB Saunders, 1990; 1230.

11 Tweedie DJ, Skilbeck CJ, Cochrane LA, *et al.* Choosing a paediatric tracheotomy tube: an update on current practice. *J Laryngol Otol* 2008; **122**: 161–9.

12 Walts PA, Murthy SC, DeCamp MM. Techniques of surgical tracheostomy. *Clin Chest Med* 2003; **24**: 413–22.

13 Palchik E, Bakken AM, Saad N, Saad WE, Davies MG. Endovascular treatment of tracheoinnominate artery fistula: a case report. *Vasc Endovascular Surg* 2007; **41**: 258–61.

Chapter 2

Elective surgical tracheotomy in the adult

Yvonne Tsui, Michael Ondik, and David Goldenberg

Case presentation

A 76-year-old patient with multiorgan failure has been intubated and ventilated in the intensive care unit (ICU) for 9 days. Of note, it was very difficult to intubate the patient. You are consulted for a tracheotomy. At physical examination, he is obese with moderately palpable cervical landmarks. Informed consent is obtained from his surrogate decision-maker. The laboratory results are checked and there is no coagulopathy. The patient is scheduled for an elective open tracheotomy in the operating room.

Introduction

A tracheotomy is a surgical procedure in which a direct airway is established by creating an opening in the anterior neck into the trachea. Three main groups of patients that benefit from elective tracheotomy: required prolonged intubation; cannot manage their airway secretions; or have an upper airway obstruction. Conversion from a translaryngeal airway to a tracheotomy minimizes patient discomfort, reduces the amount of analgesics and sedation required, and lowers the rate of long-term complications from translaryngeal airways.

Tracheotomies can improve the quality of life for patients by allowing return of speech with the use of a Passy–Muir valve [1] or a fenestrated tube, allowing oral intake, improving oral hygiene, and promoting patient mobility. A tracheotomy reduces anatomic dead space in the upper airway, decreases the work of breathing by reducing airway resistance, and increases alveolar ventilation. Better access for airway suctioning is also created for patients with unmanageable airway secretions. Tracheotomies can facilitate the weaning of ventilator-dependent patients by reducing airway resistance; this is particularly beneficial in those with borderline levels of pulmonary mechanics and high respiration rates [2].

Tracheotomy: indications

(1) *An elective tracheotomy is indicated when patients require a prolonged artificial airway.*
This group includes patients who have impaired airway protection reflexes secondary to decreased consciousness, and patients with hypoventilation secondary to central nervous system dysfunction or weakness from neuromuscular disease. The long-term complications of translaryngeal airways include glottic and subglottic stenosis, paranasal

Tracheotomy Management: A Multidisciplinary Approach, ed. Peggy A. Seidman, David Goldenberg and Elizabeth H. Sinz. Published by Cambridge University Press.

sinusitis, laryngeal injury, and vocal cord paralysis. The risk of these complications significantly increases with translaryngeal intubation beyond the 10th day [3]. Therefore, many advocate conversion to a tracheotomy early in the course of mechanical ventilation if extubation is not anticipated within 10 days.

(2) *Patients who have long-term respiratory problems or copious airway secretions can benefit from an elective tracheotomy.* Inability to clear airway secretions is an indication for tracheotomy, as it provides better access for frequent airway suctioning. Patients in this group include those with decreased bulbar muscle strength secondary to neuromuscular disease, recurrent aspiration pneumonia, and decreased levels of consciousness.

(3) *Tracheotomy can be done to bypass upper airway obstruction at or above the level of the larynx.* In the past, upper airway infections such as diphtheria, polio, tetanus, epiglottitis, and Ludwig's angina would often compromise the upper airway [4–6]. Today, maxillofacial trauma and upper airway tumors may obstruct the airway, and a tracheotomy is performed to bypass the obstruction. With inhalational injury or ingestion burn injury, edema of the oropharynx and larynx may be extensive, and may necessitate a tracheotomy. Patients with functional obstructions such as bilateral vocal cord paralysis and laryngeal edema may benefit from tracheotomies as well.

(4) Tracheotomy may be necessary for perioperative and postoperative airway management. Head and neck surgery for oral or oropharyngeal tumors can lead to extensive oropharyngeal or laryngeal edema and obstruction postoperatively. Head and neck surgeons need to plan for securing the airway in patients with complex or extensive tumor resections involving the upper airway.

Patients who have neck or severe facial traumas may require tracheotomies. Laryngeal trauma can lead to difficulty in creating or maintaining a translaryngeal airway. Endotracheal intubation in severe facial traumas can be difficult or even detrimental to the patient, and tracheotomy can be done at the discretion of the surgeon.

Contraindications

There are no absolute contraindications to open surgical tracheotomy.

Relative contraindications include active infection or burn at the tracheotomy site, poor pulmonary function, inability to transport to the operating room due to acute respiratory distress syndrome, and high peak inspiratory pressure/pulmonary artery pressure or poor oxygenation not allowing the patient to tolerate apnea.

Preoperative evaluation

Obesity, short neck, and kyphosis can change the orientation of the trachea. The cervical trachea may be shortened, or the trachea may be located entirely within the bony thorax [8]. Previous neck surgery, irradiation, or recent sternotomy can also make the neck anatomy more complex. These factors should be taken into consideration during preoperative planning. Anticoagulants and antiplatelet medications should be discontinued before a tracheotomy.

Table 2.1 Indications for tracheotomy*

Upper airway obstruction with any of the following:
Stridor
Air hunger
Retractions
Obstructive sleep apnea with documented arterial desaturation
Bilateral vocal fold paralysis
Previous neck surgery or throat trauma
Previous irradiation to the neck
Prolonged or expected prolonged intubation
Inability of patient to manage secretions, including the following:
Aspiration
Excessive bronchopulmonary secretions
Facilitation of ventilation support
Inability to intubate
Adjunct to manage head and neck surgery
Adjunct to manage significant head and neck trauma

* As defined by the American Academy of Otolaryngology-Head and Neck Surgery [7].

Operative technique

An elective surgical tracheotomy is performed in the operating room under general anesthesia. In cases where difficult intubation is anticipated an elective awake tracheotomy may be performed under local anesthesia.

The patient is positioned supine with the neck in extension aided by use of a shoulder roll. Care should be taken to avoid overextension of the neck, as this will lead to airway narrowing and low placement of the tracheotomy [9]. Monopolar electrocautery should be used with caution in a tracheotomy, as incision into the trachea will release oxygen into the surgical field raising the risk of an intraoperative fire [10].

A vertical or horizontal cutaneous incision should be made midway between the cricoid cartilage and sternal notch (Figure 2.1). A skin incision of 2–3 cm is often adequate. In obese patients, a cervical lipectomy may be performed to facilitate the procedure [11]. Care should be taken not to injure the anterior jugular vein located laterally in the surgical field. The midline raphe of the strap muscles should be identified and divided. The strap muscles are then retracted laterally. A high riding innominate artery should be determined at this point by placing one finger in the inferior aspect of the wound bed [9]. By locating the innominate artery, potential injury to the vessel and subsequent bleeding complications can be avoided.

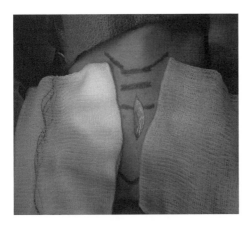

Figure 2.1 A vertical skin incision between cricoid and sternal notch.

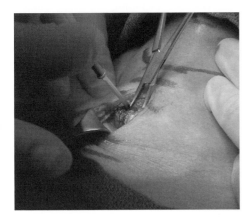

Figure 2.2 Dividing of the thyroid isthmus with a monopolar cautery.

The thyroid isthmus lies below the strap muscles, typically at the level of the third and fourth tracheal ring. The isthmus can be mobilized and retracted superiorly, or it can be divided using monopolar electrocautery if it blocks the tracheotomy site (Figure 2.2). Dividing the thyroid can prevent dislodgement of the tracheotomy tube during swallowing and decrease pressure on the anterior tracheal wall [12].

Dissection through the pretracheal fat pad should be done with care, as the inferior thyroid veins and, occasionally, the thyroid ima artery may pass through the fat pad [13]. Lateral dissection of the trachea should be minimized as the vascular supply of the trachea is located laterally and lateral dissection can risk damage to these vessels [13]. The recurrent laryngeal nerves can be damaged if the dissection extends into the tracheoesophageal groove.

Once the trachea is exposed, the cricoid cartilage should be palpated and used as a landmark. A hook should be placed below the cricoid and pulled cephalad (Figure 2.3). When it is time to make the incision into the trachea, communication between the surgical and anesthesiate is essential. The position of the endotracheal tube will need to be adjusted in concert with the procedure and the ability to ventilate may be reduced.

Adequate preoxygenation of the patient is needed, due to the apnea time during the tracheotomy and transition to tracheotomy tube ventilation. The anesthesia team should be prepared to remove the endotracheal tube by removing the circumferential wrap and. The

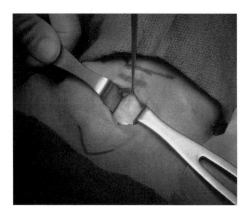

Figure 2.3 Trachea exposed, pretracheal tissue removed, note hook inserted below cricoid to stabilize and elevate trachea cephalad before making tracheotomy incision.

anesthetist should prepare to remove the endotracheal tube, including removing fixation devices. The cuff on the endotracheal tube should be deflated to avoid balloon rupture during tracheotomy, in case endotracheal ventilation is needed at a later point during the procedure. Incision of the trachea can be made between the second and third or the third and fourth tracheal rings [15].

Variations of tracheal incision that can be made:

(1) A vertical or horizontal linear incision is the simplest. With a vertical incision, tracheal stay sutures can be placed to help stabilize the trachea during the procedure. The stay sutures are positioned around the second or third tracheal ring lateral to the tracheotomy incision and placed submucosally to prevent granulation tissue formation. They may be left in place postoperatively and taped to the anterior chest wall until the first tracheotomy tube change. The stay sutures can be used to pull the trachea anteriorly during a tube change or reinsertion in the event of inadvertent decannulation.

(2) A Björk flap, which is an inferiorly based trapdoor flap, can also be used (Figure 2.4). It is created by making two vertical incisions that form the lateral borders of the tracheotomy, and the superior aspect of the incisions are joined with a horizontal incision. The flap is reflected anteriorly and sewn to the inferior aspect of the tracheotomy wound. The flap suture can be released once the tract has started to mature, usually 3–5 days postoperatively. The advantage of using a Björk flap is that it draws the trachea anteriorly and closer to the skin, allowing easier access to the tracheotomy and facilitating tube replacements.

(3) A tracheal window can be created by removing a round or vertical oval portion of the anterior trachea. This can be done using a tracheotomy punch [16,17], scalpel, or scissors (Figure 2.5). The window generally spans from the mid-portion of the third tracheal ring to the mid-portion of the fourth tracheal ring.

After the tracheotomy is made, the endotracheal tube is withdrawn by the anesthetist until the tip is above the incision. A range of tracheotomy tube sizes should be available in the operating room. The tube should be chosen based on the size of the patient's trachea. A pre-chosen tracheotomy tube along with its obturator is inserted into the trachea, and the obturator is removed. The inner cannula of the tube is inserted, the cuff is inflated, and ventilation via the tracheotomy tube is initiated. Proper placement of the tube is confirmed

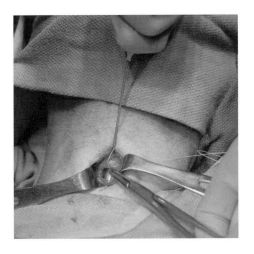

Figure 2.4 Tracheotomy window formed, using Björk flap.

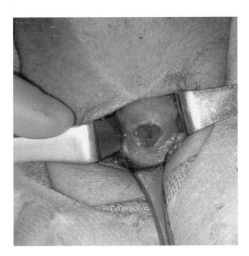

Figure 2.5 Tracheotomy window formed with tracheotomy punch, endotracheal tube can be viewed through window (courtesy of David Eisle MD).

with bilateral auscultation and detection of end-tidal CO_2. Once adequate ventilation with the tracheotomy is confirmed, the endotracheal tube can be removed. The tracheotomy tube is secured to the anterior neck with four sutures, one at each corner of the flange. It is suggested that a collar be used to secure the tube further.

Tracheotomy tube selection

A tracheotomy tube should accommodate the patient's functional needs and conform to the anatomy of the airway. Proper tube selection will minimize discomfort and avoid damage to the tracheal wall. Tracheotomy tubes have varying inner diameters, outer diameters, lengths, and curvatures.

Tracheotomy tubes can be standard length, as well as extra length. Extra length tubes with extra proximal or extra distal lengths are available. Extra proximal length tubes have longer horizontal length and are appropriate for patients with larger necks. Extra distal length tubes can facilitate placement in patients with tracheal abnormalities.

Tracheotomy tubes can be curved or angled, and a tube that best conforms to the shape of the trachea should be chosen. A curved tube may not fit patients perfectly, as the trachea is straight. An angled tube has a curved portion and a straight portion. As the tracheal portion of the tube is straight, an angled tube will minimize trauma and pressure to the tracheal wall.

Tracheotomy tubes can be cuffed or uncuffed. Cuffed tubes have the advantage of providing some protection from aspiration, and more effective positive pressure ventilation. Minimal occluding cuff pressures should be used to minimize tracheal mucosal injury.

Postoperative care

Patients who have undergone a tracheotomy are monitored in an intermediate or intensive care setting overnight, with continuous pulse oximetry monitoring. Frequent dressing changes should be performed in the immediate postoperative period, as secretions can accumulate around the tracheotomy site. Constant humidification of inhaled air should be provided to prevent crust formation at the site of the incision. Suctioning of the tracheotomy tube, as well as cleaning of the inner cannula, needs to be performed frequently to prevent the buildup of mucus plugs.

The first tracheotomy tube change, if necessary, is performed on postoperative days 5–7. This allows enough time for the tract to mature.

Decannulation

Before decannulation, the tracheotomy tube is gradually downsized and capped for 24 h. If the patient demonstrates satisfactory ventilation with a capped tracheotomy tube, decannulation may proceed.

Complications

The rate of significant complications from tracheotomies in recent studies was reported to be as low as 4.3% among adults, with a mortality rate of 0.7%. The most common complications include hemorrhage, obstruction, and inadvertent decannulation. Mortality is most often secondary to hemorrhage or inadvertent decannulation [18].

Bleeding intraoperatively or postoperatively is the most common complication from tracheotomies. Sites of bleeding include the anterior jugular vein, and thyroid. Bleeding may not be evident until the postoperative period, with increased venous pressure secondary to coughing or changes in cardiovascular parameters. Minor bleeding can be controlled by light packing or the application of dressings. Severe bleeding warrants exploration and ligation or cauterization of vessels. Injury to the innominate artery in the anterior trachea can lead to life-threatening hemorrhage.

Tube obstruction in the early postoperative period is most likely secondary to blood clots, tube impingement on the posterior tracheal wall, or tube displacement. Obstructions occurring later in the course as the stoma matures can be due to mucus plugs or granulation tissue.

Inadvertent decannulation is a serious complication that can arise in the early postoperative period. The reported rate of inadvertent decannulation among tracheotomies is 1% among adults [19], which are lower than accidental decannulation rates of endotracheal intubation. Inadvertent decannulation can lead to respiratory distress and patient death if

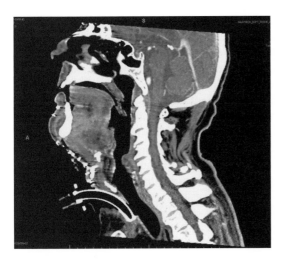

Figure 2.6 False route caused by reinsertion of displaced tracheotomy tube.

an airway is not secured promptly. Factors affecting rates of inadvertent decannulation include the length of the tube, thickness of the neck, location of the tracheotomy site, postoperative swelling, and method of securing the tube. Patients at higher risk of decannulation are obese and are moved at a higher frequency, such as those with pressure ulcers. To avoid inadvertent decannulation, the tracheotomy tube should be secured to the patient's neck. In the event that a patient is inadvertently decannulated, securing an airway immediately is a priority. Although it is possible to reinsert the tube at the tracheotomy site, poor visualization can lead to misplacement and creation of false passages in the anterior neck (Figure 2.6). If direct insertion of the tracheotomy tube is attempted, it should be limited to one or two attempts. If direct insertion fails an airway needs to be re-established urgently – transoral reintubation should be considered. A tracheotomy tube may be replaced electively later on.

A tracheotomy is considered a clean-contaminated wound. Infection is a rare complication, as the wound is left open to facilitate drainage of secretions. However, improper handling of tracheal secretions may lead to local infections; therefore, strict local hygiene should be observed. Mucosal injury can contribute to the development of tracheitis and stomal cellulitis, which must be treated promptly to prevent complications such as tracheal stenosis. Infections can be treated with antibiotics and local wound care. Antibiotics are only indicated with signs of infections, and prophylactic antibiotics are not necessary. More severe infections such as necrotizing fasciitis, clavicular osteomyelitis, and mediastinitis are exceedingly rare, but have been reported [20].

Pneumothorax and pneumomediastinum are rare complications of tracheotomy, and can occur because of excessive pretracheal tissue dissection or misplacement of the tracheotomy tube. Subcutaneous emphysema, pneumothorax, and pneumomediastinum can be prevented by proper surgical technique, minimizing the amount of dissection along the tissue planes and ensuring that the trachea is exposed sufficiently before incision into the trachea. Reducing the negative inspiratory force with an endotracheal airway intraoperatively can reduce the incidence of air dissection along facial planes. Some surgeons order a chest X-ray postoperatively to confirm proper tube placement.

Tracheal stenosis may be a long-term complication of tracheotomy. Stenosis most commonly occurs at the location of the tube cuff and at the tracheotomy stoma. One mechanism of injury leading to tracheal stenosis is thought to be mucosal ischemia secondary to high cuff pressures [21]. The elevated pressure levels lead to tracheal ulcerations that heal with granulation tissue formation and fibrosis, thereby narrowing the airway. A second mechanism of injury is the disruption to the tracheal cartilage caused by the tracheotomy tube, which can lead to instability of the trachea and further tissue damage. This causes stenosis at the level of the stoma. Risk factors for tracheal stenosis include advanced age, hypotension, infection, neoplasm, gastroesophageal reflux, elevated cuff pressures, and duration of cannulation. Patients with stenosis can remain asymptomatic until the lumen diameter has been reduced by 50–75%. Presenting symptoms of tracheal stenosis include dyspnea, cough, and inability to clear secretions. Stenosis can be treated with endoscopic excision, endoscopic dilations, carbon dioxide laser resection, or steroid injections. Longer lesions can be treated with resection of the stenotic segment and repaired with end-to-end anastomosis.

Tracheoinnominate fistulas are the most lethal of complications and can occur when the tip of the tube or the cuff itself erodes through the anterior wall of the trachea into the innominate artery. Risk factors include a high innominate artery or a tracheotomy located lower in the neck. Tracheoinnominate fistulas manifest as bleeding from the tracheotomy site, and can be life threatening if the innominate artery ruptures. Although a rare complication, the mortality rate of tracheoinnominate fistulas approaches 90% [22–27]. Two-thirds of tracheoinnominate fistulas occur within the first 3 weeks after a tracheotomy [28], but they can still arise years after the procedure [29,30]. A sentinel bleed can precede massive hemorrhage, and warrants immediate fiberoptic tracheal examination [31] and immediate surgical repair is indicated.

Tracheoesophageal fistula results from erosion of the tracheotomy tube or cuff into the posterior tracheal wall, caused by an overinflated cuff or an improperly fitted cuffed tube sometimes combined with an indwelling nasogastric tube. Common presentations include chronic cough, aspiration of tube feeds, aspiration pneumonia, or gastric distention with air. Barium swallow or endoscopic evaluation can confirm the diagnosis. Surgical repair of the tracheoesophageal fistula is necessary, as it is associated with mortality rates as high as 70–80% [32].

Tracheomalacia is the loss of tracheal cartilage, resulting in excessive airway compliance. Airway ischemia due to high cuff pressures can cause chondritis and destruction of the cartilage [33]. Endoscopically, findings of a widened posterior wall with expiratory collapse is characteristic of tracheomalacia [33,34]. Severity of symptoms can vary, and tracheoplasty may be required in severe cases.

Conclusions

Tracheotomy is one of the most commonly performed procedures in critically ill patients. Indications for tracheotomies include requirement for long-term intubation, inability to clear airway secretions, upper airway obstruction, and severe facial and neck trauma. Tracheotomies can improve the quality of life for patients requiring long-term intubation. Early conversion from a translaryngeal airway to a tracheotomy can prevent complications from prolonged intubation. Patient factors such as morbid obesity, kyphosis, previous neck surgery, or irradiation can cause variations in neck anatomy; these factors should be taken into consideration during planning. In selecting a tracheotomy tube, one that best conforms to the patient's anatomy should be chosen. Complications from tracheotomies can be minimized by proper surgical technique and postoperative care.

References

1. Passy V, Prentice W, Darnell-Neal R. Passy-Muir tracheostomy speaking valve on ventilator-dependent patients. *Laryngoscope* 1993; **103**: 653–8.

2. Heffner JE. The role of tracheotomy in weaning. *Chest* 2001; **120**: 477–81.

3. Whited RE. A prospective study of laryngotracheal sequelae in long-term intubation. *Laryngoscope* 1984; **94**: 365–77.

4. Mallampati SR, *et al*. A clinical sign to predict difficult tracheal intubation: a prospective study. *Can Anaesth Soc J* 1985; **32**: 429–34.

5. Samsoon GL, Young JR. Difficult tracheal intubation: a retrospective study. *Anaesthesia* 1987; **42**: 487–90.

6. Wenig BL, Applebaum EL. Indications for and techniques of tracheotomy. *Clin Chest Med* 1997; **12**: 545–53.

7. Archer SM, Baugh RF, Nelms CR. *2000 Clinical Indicators Compendium* 45. Alexandria, VA: American Academy of Otolaryngology-Head and Neck Surgery, 2000.

8. Grillo HC. *General Thoracic Surgery*. 5th edn. Lippincott Williams & Wilkins, 2000.

9. Scurry WC, McGinn JD. Operative tracheotomy. *Oper Tech Otolaryngol Head Neck Surg* 2007; **18**: 85–9.

10. Aly A, McIlwain M, Duncavage JA. Electrosurgery-induced endotracheal tube ignition during tracheotomy. *Ann Otol Rhinol Laryngol* 1991; **100**: 31–3.

11. Gross ND, Cohen JI, Andersen PE, Wax MK. "Defatting" tracheotomy in morbidly obese patients. *Laryngoscope* 2002; **112**: 1940–4.

12. Kirchner JA. Avoiding problems in tracheotomy. *Laryngoscope* 1986; **96**: 55–7.

13. Allan MS. Surgical anatomy of the trachea. *Chest Surg Clin N Am* 1996; **6**: 72–81.

14. Weber AL, Grillo HC. Tracheal stenosis: an analysis of 151 cases. *Radiol Clin North Am* 1978; **16**: 291–308.

15. Chalian AA. In: Wiley WS, DW Wilmore DW, eds. *ACS Surgery: Principles and Practice*. BC Decker Inc., 2009.

16. Goldenberg D, Bhatti N. In: Cummings CW, ed. *Cummings: Otolaryngology: Head and Neck Surgery*, 4th edn. Mosby, Inc., 2005.

17. Mitchell R, Eisle D, Goldenberg D. Tracheotomy punch for urgent tracheotomy. *Laryngoscope* 2010; **120**(4): 745–8.

18. Goldenberg, D. *et al*. Tracheotomy complications: a retrospective stufy of 1130 cases. *Otolaryngol Head Neck Surg* 2000; **123**: 495–500.

19. Reibel JF. Tracheostomy/tracheotomy. *Respir Care* 1999; **44**: 820–3.

20. Wang RC, Perlman PW, Parnes SM. Near-fatal complications of tracheotomy infections and their prevention. *Head Neck* 1989; **11**: 528–33.

21. Stauffer JL, Olson DE, Petty TL. Complications and consequences of endotracheal intubation and tracheotomy: a prospective study of 150 critically ill adult patients. *Am J Med* 1981; **70**: 65–76.

22. Nelems JM. Tracheo-innominate artery fistula. *Am J Surg* 1981; **141**: 526–7.

23. Jones JW, Reynolds M, Hewitt RL, Drapanas T. Tracheo-innominate artery erosion: successful mangement of a devasting complication. *Ann Surg* 1976; **184**: 194–204.

24. Cooper JD. Tracheo-innominate artery fistula. *Ann Thorac Surg* 1977; **24**: 439–57.

25. Arola MK, Ingberg M, Sotarauta M., Vanttinen E. Tracheo-arterial erosion complicating tracheostomy. *Ann Chir Gynaecol Fenn* 1979; **68**: 9–17.

26. Bloss RS, Ward RE. Survival after tracheo-innominate artery fistula. *Am J Surg* 1980; **140**: 251–3.

27. Weiss JB, Ozment KL, Westbrook KC. Tracheo-innominate artery fistula after repair of tracheal stenosis: problem and prevention. *J Thorac Cardiovasc Surg* 1974; **69**: 430–2.

28. Tournigand P, Djurakdjian S, Jajah S, Morisset P. Successful surgical repair of a tracheo innominate fistula: tactical considerations. *J Cardiovasc Surg (Torino)* 1982; **23**: 247–51.

29. Ridley RW, Zwischenberger JB. Tracheoinnominate fistula: surgical management of an iatrogenic disaster. *J Laryngol Otol* 2006; **120**: 676–80.

30. Sawamura, Y. *et al.* Surgical repair for tracheo-innominate artery fistula with a muscle flap. *Jpn J Thorac Cardiovasc Surg* 2003; **51**: 630–3.

31. Deslauriers J, Ginsberg RJ, Nelems JM, Pearson FG. Innominate artery rupture. A major complication of tracheal surgery. *Ann Thorac Surg* 1975; **20**: 671–7.

32. Thomas AN. Management of tracheoesophageal fistula caused by cuffed tracheal tubes. *Am J Surg* 1972; **124**: 181–9.

33. Feist JH, Johnson TH, Wilson RJ. Acquired tracheomalacia: etiology and differential diagnosis. *Chest* 1975; **68**: 340–5.

34. Sue RD, Susanto I. Long-term complications of artificial airways. *Clin Chest Med* 2003; **24**: 457–71.

Percutaneous tracheotomy

Garret Choby, Dmitri Bezinover, and David Goldenberg

Case presentation

An older man with multiple broken ribs and lung injury has been intubated and ventilated in the intensive care unit of a busy urban hospital for 12 days. Although it is clear that he should undergo a tracheotomy, operating room time is at a premium, and he has been "bumped" from the schedule several times due to cases that are more urgent and other surgeries that have gone on longer than originally scheduled. His case is elective, but it is increasingly apparent that a tracheotomy will let him proceed to the next phase of his care and it should be performed sooner rather than later.

Introduction

Interest in a percutaneous approach to tracheotomies first began in 1955 when Shelden *et al.* performed the first modern percutaneous tracheotomy (PT) [1]. The complication rate, however, was very high due to traumatic lacerations of surrounding structures by the trocar [2–4]. Thus, safer and more efficient methods continued to be developed.

In 1985, Ciaglia *et al.* used an innovative technique based upon serial dilations with sequentially larger dilators placed over a needle guidewire [5]. The development of this technique was the culmination of an increased interest in minimally invasive procedures, technological advances, and an increased emphasis on time and cost constraints.

With this initial innovative technique, the PT has gained widespread acceptance in intensive care units and operating rooms across the world. Additionally, multiple variations of the Seldinger technique have evolved, including the use of dilating forceps, screw-action dilators, and a translaryngeal approach. The consistent feature of all these techniques is the use of the Seldinger guidewire to provide a safe, controlled approach to dilation of the tracheal opening. In expert hands, the entire procedure usually takes 5–10 min, and rarely longer than 15 min. Additionally, the low cost of the percutaneous approach initially led to its rise in popularity in the United States and elsewhere [6].

Indications

Indications for PT are identical to those of the standard open tracheotomy. The most common is the need for prolonged endotracheal intubation and mechanical ventilation during respiratory failure [7]. Other indications include airway obstruction from foreign bodies, laryngeal

Tracheotomy Management: A Multidisciplinary Approach, ed. Peggy A. Seidman,
David Goldenberg and Elizabeth H. Sinz. Published by Cambridge University Press.
© Cambridge University Press 2011.

Table 3.1 Indication for percutaneous tracheotomy

Indications for percutaneous tracheotomy
Need for prolonged intubation for respiratory failure

Airway obstruction
  Foreign body
  Neoplasm
  Laryngeal trauma
  Bilateral vocal cord paralysis
  Congenital airway lesions (vascular web, laryngeal hypoplasia)

Prophylaxis for extensive head and neck procedures
Severe sleep apnea *refractory* to medical therapy (continuous positive airway pressure) or less invasive surgical procedures

trauma, neoplasm, bilateral vocal cord paralysis, or edema. Specific reasons may also include severe sleep apnea and extensive head and neck procedures [7–9] (Table 3.1).

Tracheotomy is beneficial in decreasing dead space and reducing airway resistance when compared with intubation. In critically ill patients, a small difference in airway resistance may play a key role in weaning a patient in mechanical ventilation [10]. Some experts argue that other significant advantages of tracheotomy include improved ability to remove secretions, enhanced oral hygiene, and less laryngeal damage than other techniques [11,12]. Moreover, all of these improvements help make the patient more comfortable than an endotracheal tube.

Contraindications and limitations

Although PT has gained widespread use, recognizing the contraindications is imperative. Absolute contraindications include the need for an emergent airway or inability to intubate the patient. Pre-adolescent patients are also not appropriate candidates for PT [7,9].

Relative contraindications include thyroid mass, poorly demarcated or obstructed landmarks, or severe coagulopathy (INR > 1.5 or platelets < 50 000). Evidence of infection at or near the PT site should also preclude a percutaneous approach. Morbid obesity, previously considered a relative contraindication, may be overcome and there are now specific PT kits for use in these patients (Figure 3.1).

Additional considerations must be taken into account to ensure the safety of the patient. PT generally should not be carried out in patients in whom a difficult reintubation is anticipated or in patients with positive end-expiratory pressure > 15 cm H_2O, peak airway pressure > 45 mmHg, or PaO_2/FiO_2 < 200 [9,13].

Preoperative workup

In general, a coagulation panel and complete blood count are obtained before the procedure to assess bleeding risk. Platelets should be > 50 000 and bleeding time < 10 min. Additionally, the patient's oxygenation status should be closely monitored during surgery with a pulse oximeter [14].

Techniques for percutaneous tracheotomy

All current PT methods are based upon the Seldinger technique of dilators placed over a guide-wire [3]. It is recommended that PT be performed under simultaneous video bronchoscopy [15].

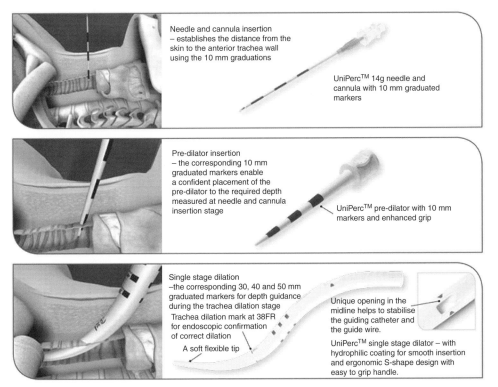

Needle and cannula insertion
– establishes the distance from the skin to the anterior trachea wall using the 10 mm graduations

UniPerc™ 14g needle and cannula with 10 mm graduated markers

Pre-dilator insertion
– the corresponding 10 mm graduated markers enable a confident placement of the pre-dilator to the required depth measured at needle and cannula insertion stage

UniPerc™ pre-dilator with 10 mm markers and enhanced grip

Single stage dilation
–the corresponding 30, 40 and 50 mm graduated markers for depth guidance during the trachea dilation stage
Trachea dilation mark at 38FR for endoscopic confirmation of correct dilation
A soft flexible tip

Unique opening in the midline helps to stabilise the guiding catheter and the guide wire.
UniPerc™ single stage dilator – with hydrophilic coating for smooth insertion and ergonomic S-shape design with easy to grip handle.

Figure 3.1 UniPerc, a percutaneous dilational tracheotomy kit produced by Portex. (Courtesy of Smiths Medical, Keene, New Hampshire, USA.)

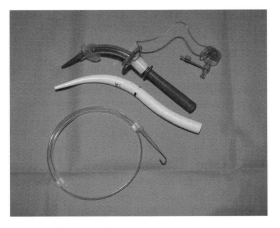

Figure 3.2 Ciaglia single dilator percutaneous dilational tracheotomy.

Ciaglia method (percutaneous dilating technique)

The Ciaglia method of PT has become one of the most popular techniques in the USA (Figure 3.2).

The patient should be positioned with a shoulder roll to allow moderate extension of his or her neck. Landmarks should be palpated and marked on the patient's skin (Figure 3.3).

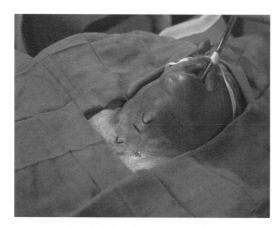

Figure 3.3 The patient's cervical landmarks should be identified a shoulder roll placed and the patient prepped and draped.

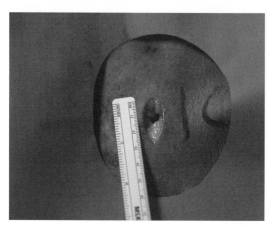

Figure 3.4 A small skin incision (either horizontal or vertical) is made between the cricoid and the sternal notch.

The neck is prepped and the area draped in the usual sterile fashion. Lidocaine 1% with 1:100 000 epinephrine is infiltrated locally. The initial incision may be made vertically or horizontally along the midline at the level of the inferior border of the cricoid cartilage (Figure 3.4). The typical incision is about 2–3 cm in length. Dissection of the pretracheal tissue is performed to push the thyroid isthmus inferiorly. At this stage, bronchoscopic visualization of the tracheal lumen is carried out to allow visualization of the remainder of the procedure (Figure 3.5). The tip of the bronchoscope may be flexed 90 degrees, close to the anterior wall of the trachea, to fully transilluminate it through the overlying soft tissue (Figure 3.6).

Following site selection, the introducer needle of the cannula is advanced along the inferior edge of the light reflex through the anterior tracheal membrane with care to avoid advancing the needle into the posterior tracheal wall [7,14] (Figure 3.7). The needle is then withdrawn while the cannula is maintained within the lumen of the trachea. A J-tipped guidewire is then introduced through the cannula (Figure 3.8). The cannula is removed. The dilator is inserted over the guidewire and advanced through the anterior wall of the trachea (Figure 3.9). Following dilation, a tracheotomy tube is placed over the guidewire and advanced towards the trachea. After placement of the tracheotomy tube, the guidewire is removed and the cuff of the tracheotomy tube is inflated; CO_2 return is confirmed by continuous waveform capnography [6,7]. The tube should be secured with four non-absorbable sutures and a tracheotomy collar.

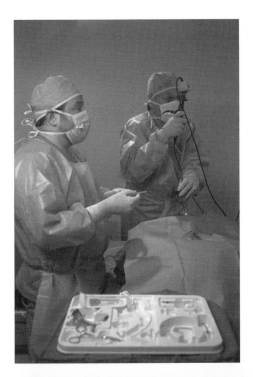

Figure 3.5 Simultaneous bronchoscopy during placement of percutaneous tracheotomy.

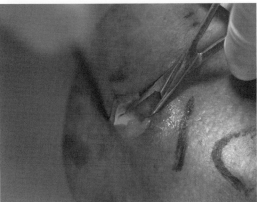

Figure 3.6 Bronchoscopic transillumination of the anterior tracheal wall seen through skin incision.

Griggs technique (guidewire dilating forceps technique)

The Griggs technique differs in its use of guidewire dilator forceps (GWDF) as opposed to the serial dilators or one-step dilator of the Ciaglia technique [16]. In a similar fashion, it also makes use of the Seldinger guidewire. The GWDF has a curved design, which reduces the risk of damage to the posterior tracheal wall upon insertion (Figure 3.10).

The role of the GWDF is to enlarge the hole in the anterior wall of the trachea to allow placement of the tracheotomy tube. The initial part of the procedure is similar to the Ciaglia technique, as described above, including positioning and incision [9].

At this point, a 14-gauge intravenous needle and cannula with attached syringe is inserted along the midline incision and advanced until air bubbles back into the syringe, confirming

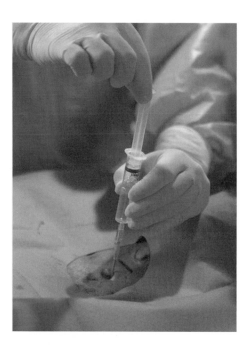

Figure 3.7 Insertion of catheter over needle into trachea. Note aspiration of bubbles into liquid confirms placement of needle into trachea.

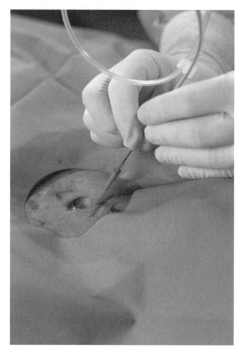

Figure 3.8 Insertion of guidewire through catheter into trachea.

placement in the trachea. The needle is retracted while the cannula remains in place. The J-tipped Seldinger wire is then introduced into the trachea through the cannula. The cannula is removed leaving the guidewire in place. The tip of the wire is then passed through the bore at the end of the closed GWDF to advance through the soft tissues of the anterior neck. The

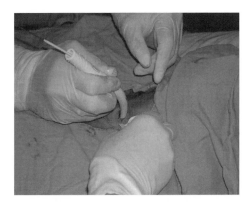

Figure 3.9 Insertion of Ciaglia single dilator over guidewire into trachea (figure courtesy of Dr. Jorge A. Ramirez).

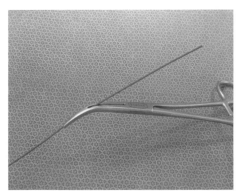

Figure 3.10 Griggs guidewire dilating forceps technique.

forceps handles are lifted vertically to allow penetration into the anterior wall of the trachea and advanced such that the tip lies longitudinally within the trachea. The GWDF is then opened to dilate the tracheotomy in the anterior tracheal wall (Figure 3.11). After withdrawing the forceps, the tracheotomy tube is placed over the guidewire and advanced into the trachea (Figure 3.12). Carbon dioxide return is confirmed by capnography. The cuff is inflated appropriately and the tube secured with non-absorbable sutures and a tracheotomy collar [9,13,17].

Fantoni's technique (translaryngeal approach)

The translaryngeal approach for tracheotomies was first described by Fantoni *et al.* in 1997 [18]. After positioning and draping has occurred, as previously described, the endotracheal tube is moved back to the glottic area under vision by direct laryngoscopy. A flexible bronchoscope is then advanced through this endotracheal tube to allow visualization of the tracheal lumen. A needle is inserted into the anterior trachea and a Seldinger guidewire retrogradely advanced upwards in the trachea and out of the patient's mouth. A unique device composed of a flexible plastic cone with metal tip attached to an armored tracheal cannula is attached to the guidewire and advanced through the oral cavity and into the trachea.

Once the cannula reaches the site of the intratracheal guidewire piercing the anterior trachea, moderate force is applied anteriorly on the cone and cannula by the operator to penetrate the tracheal wall [19]. Simultaneous counter-pressure is held on the anterior neck by the operator's other hand, ensuring maximal control. Once the metal tip has emerged at the skin, the cone is advanced to its final placement [19,20].

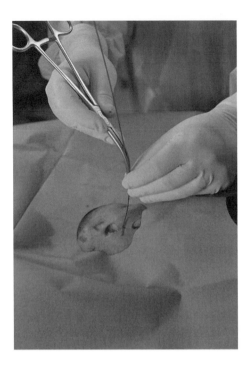

Figure 3.11 Griggs guidewire dilating forceps technique – specialized Griggs forceps being threaded over guidewire.

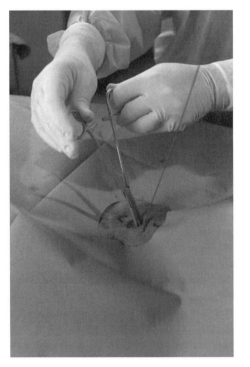

Figure 3.12 Griggs guidewire dilating forceps technique – dilation of trachea with forceps.

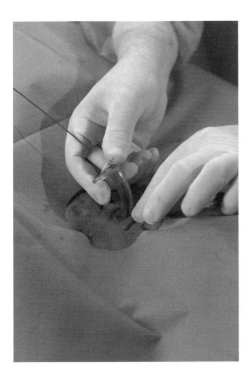

Figure 3.13 Percutaneous tracheotomy tube inserted over guidewire.

Soft tissue trauma is minimized by stabilization of the anterior trachea and careful application of counterforce, as the metal tip and cone are advanced through the anterior trachea [20].

PercTwist (screw-action dilator)

The PercTwist is a screw-action dilator, developed to address the problem of excessive force exerted on the tracheal wall that has plagued traditional PT techniques. The concept underlying its development is the avoidance of excessive downward force on the trachea by using a screw-action that lifts the trachea upwards on the dilating device, as opposed to forcing the dilator downwards into the trachea. The procedure proceeds with insertion of the needle and guidewire. Instead of the use of serial dilators, the PercTwist is inserted over the guidewire to the level of the trachea. It is advanced with a rotational action, which lifts the trachea upwards instead of exerting pressure downwards. The remainder of the procedure proceeds in a parallel manner to the aforementioned Ciaglia technique [4,21,22].

Anesthesia considerations

It is crucial that an experienced person administers the necessary sedative hypnotics and monitors physiologic parameters. Advanced skills in airway management are extremely valuable when unanticipated complications or difficulties arise. The patient is mechanically ventilated for approximately 5 min before the start of the procedure with the fraction of inspired oxygen at 1.0. Blood pressure, heart rate, respiratory rate, and pulse oximetry are monitored throughout [17].

Two important issues specific to PT that may arise during the course of the procedure are accidental penetration of the endotracheal tube cuff with the introducer needle during initial puncture of the anterior tracheal wall and possible dislocation of the endotracheal tube.

To resolve such issues quickly, it is crucial there is clear communication between the physicians performing the procedure and monitoring the physiologic parameters of the patient.

Postoperative complications

Short- and long-term complications of PTs have been well described in the literature. The most common immediate complication is bleeding. Goldenberg *et al.* studied the outcomes of 75 patients undergoing PT with the Griggs technique and reported stomal cellulitis (one case), subcutaneous emphysema (one), and hemorrhage (two) [9,13]. In another study, Kumar *et al.* demonstrated that of 36 patients, one had postoperative bleeding and two developed wound infection within 1 week of the procedure [23]. Other rare short-term complications include pneumothorax, esophageal injury, and tracheal wall penetration [9].

Long-term complications have been reported extensively in a number of studies and meta-analyses. A study by Steele and co-workers followed up patients with spiral computed tomography scan and demonstrated tracheal dilation in eight of 25 patients and no cases of stenosis. They reported voice change as the most common complaint occurring in 11 of 25 patients [24]. In addition, Sviri and colleagues found the most common complications in their patient population were voice change (38%) and chronic severe cough (12%). Additionally, eight of 41 patients (19.5%) had obstruction based upon spirometry but only two were symptomatic with stridor or shortness of breath (5%) [25]. Another study demonstrated 34 of 38 patients (89.5%) developed tracheal stenosis but less than 25% were symptomatic and only one of 38 experienced clinically relevant stenosis. It has also been reported that this stenosis was dependent upon the puncture site and tracheal ring fracture while inserting the dilator. Consequently, this group advocated careful dilation under endoscopic guidance [9,26].

In 2007, Higgins and Punthakee published a large meta-analysis of 15 prospective trials including 973 patients [27]. In their analysis, they demonstrated the most common long-term complications were decannulation/obstruction, minor hemorrhage, wound infection, unfavorable scarring, and subglottic stenosis. There was no significant difference in these complication rates between open and percutaneous techniques [27].

A number of issues relating to PT are currently under debate. Simultaneous bronchoscopic visualization during PT has traditionally been a point of controversy, although it is generally accepted as the modern standard of care with >90% of intensive care units currently using it regularly [28,29]. Intraoperative use of bronchoscopy allows clear visualization of the initial needle insertion to improve precision of placement. The most significant advantage is prevention of injury to the posterior tracheal wall during initial insertion of needle, guidewire, and dilators. The use of bronchoscopy is not without its drawbacks. It may contribute to oxygen desaturation and retention of CO_2 during the procedure and thus could be contraindicated in patients who cannot tolerate elevated CO_2 levels (e.g., traumatic brain injury) [9,30]. It should be noted that this traditional notion is unlikely to be clinically significant. As reported by Kost in 2005 in a series of 500 consecutive patients undergoing PT with bronchoscopic guidance, the potential complications associated with simultaneous use of bronchoscopy pale in comparison with its benefits [15]. Only 14 of 500 patients (2.8%) experienced transient oxygen desaturation. Within this article, the overall complication rate in non-endoscopic cases was 233 of 1385 patients (16.8%) compared with 71 complications of 851 patients (8.3%) in endoscopically guided cases. This difference was statistically significant ($P < 0.0001$) [15].

Another important consideration is increased intracranial pressure (ICP) present in many of these critically ill patients. A patient with an acute rise in ICP is not a good candidate for tracheotomy, but if their ICP is stable before the PT procedure, they can be continually monitored throughout with an ICP monitor. If elevated ICP is noted, increasing sedation can frequently resolve this issue. Other factors may help, such as increasing ventilation to decrease the CO_2 level, and administering mannitol.

The debate of open versus percutaneous approaches to tracheotomy has been widely discussed. Percutaneous techniques were originally developed out of an interest in minimally invasive procedures that could be performed outside of the operating room with minimal personnel and cost. It is generally held that the percutaneous technique is as safe as the open technique in properly selected patients. PT requires fewer personnel, less time, and less money [6].

Overall, rates of significant hemorrhage have been shown to be less common with PT when compared with standard tracheotomy. A large retrospective study of 794 patients with standard open tracheotomy by Arola showed that bloody secretions occurred in 22% of patients and that a catastrophic complication, tracheoarterial fistula, occurred in 0.6% of the cohort [31]. A meta-analysis by Cheng and Fee in 2000 compared outcomes in PT versus standard tracheotomy, demonstrating that PT produced less intraoperative minor bleeding (9% versus 25%), less postoperative bleeding (7% versus 18%), and resulted in fewer overall complications (14% versus 60%) [32].

There is a well-described learning curve that exists with PT, i.e., technical aspects of the procedure may be difficult to master by an inexperienced physician. There is an active debate concerning how young physicians should be trained, but is difficult to evaluate fully the relative safety and efficacy between the two approaches because many existing studies lack a rigorous design. Ideally, physicians in training should receive instruction in both open and percutaneous techniques [6].

It is interesting to note the relative differences in approach to PT that exist internationally. According to a 2006 nationwide survey of 455 adult intensive care units in Germany, tracheotomy was cited as their most commonly performed procedure. Moreover, this survey found that 328 (73%) of responders chose PT as the procedure of choice with only 54 (12%) selecting surgical tracheotomy [28].

Conclusions

To update the case report at the beginning, the intensivist and surgeon arrange with the nursing staff and respiratory therapist to perform a percutaneous tracheotomy at the patient's bedside in the ICU. The procedure is completed in about 15 min.

References

1. Shelden CH, Pudenz RH, Freshwater DB, et al. New method for tracheotomy. J Neurosurg 1955; **12**: 428–31.

2. Goldenberg D, Golz A, Netzer A, et al. Tracheotomy: changing indications and a review of 1,130 cases. J Otolaryngol 2002; **31**: 211–15.

3. Seldinger SI. Catheter replacement of the needle in percutaneous arteriography. Acta Radiol 1953; **39**: 368–76.

4. Durbin C. Techniques for performing tracheostomy. Respir Care 2005; **50**(4): 488–96.

5. Ciaglia P, Firsching R, Syniec C. Elective percutaneous dilatational tracheostomy: a new simple bedside procedure; preliminary report. Chest 1985; **87**(6): 715–19.

6. Susanato I. Comparing percutaneous tracheostomy with open surgical tracheostomy: both will coexist until robust evidence becomes available. BMJ 2002; **324**: 3–4.

7. Bhatti N. Percutaneous dilational tracheotomy: Ciaglia method. In: Goldenberg D, Friedman M, eds. Operative

Techniques in Head and Neck Surgery. New York: Elsevier, 2007; 18: 90–4.

8.   Scurry W, McGinn J. Operative tracheotomy. In: Goldenberg D, Friedman M, eds. *Operative Techniques in Head and Neck Surgery.* New York: Elsevier, 2007; 18: 90–4.

9.   Park S, Goldenberg D. Percutaneous tracheotomy: Griggs technique. In: Goldenberg D, Friedman M, eds. *Operative Techniques in Head and Neck Surgery.* New York: Elsevier, 2007; 18: 95–8.

10.   Pierson D. Tracheostomy and weaning. *Respir Care* 2005; 50(4): 526–33.

11.   Jaeger J, Littlewood K, Durbin C. The role of tracheostomy in weaning from mechanical ventilation. *Respir Care* 2002; 47(4): 469–80.

12.   Hsu C, Chen K, Chang C, *et al.* Timing of tracheostomy as a determinant of weaning success in critically ill patients: a retrospective study. *Crit Care* 2005; 9: 46–52.

13.   Goldenberg D, Golz A, Huri A, *et al.* Percutaneous dilation tracheotomy versus surgical tracheotomy: our experience. *Otolaryngol Head Neck Surg* 2003; 128: 358–63.

14.   Westphal K, Byhahn C, Hans-Joachim W, Lischke V. Percutaneous tracheostomy: a clinical comparison of dilational (Ciaglia) and translaryngeal (Fantoni) techniques. *Anesth Analg* 1999; 89: 938–43.

15.   Kost K. Endoscopic percutaneous dilational tracheotomy: a perspective evaluation of 500 consecutive cases. *Laryngoscope* 2005; 115: 1–30.

16.   Griggs WM, Worthley LI, Gilligan JE, Thomas PD, Myburg JA. A simple percutaneous tracheostomy technique. *Surg Gynecol Obstet* 1990; 170(6): 543–5.

17.   Sharp D, Castellanos P. Clinical outcomes of bedside percutaneous dilational tracheostomy with suspension laryngoscopy for airway control. *Ann Otol Rhinol Laryngol* 2009; 118(2): 98–9.

18.   Fantoni A, Ripamonti D. A non-derivative, non-surgical tracheostomy: the translaryngeal method. *Intensive Care Med* 1997; 23(4): 386–92.

19.   Fantoni A, Ripamonti D, Lesmo A, Zanoni CI. Translaryngeal tracheostomy. A new era? *Minerva Anestesiol* 1996; 62(10): 313–25.

20.   Meininger D, Byhahn C. Translaryngeal tracheotomy. In: Goldenberg D, Friedman M, eds. *Operative Techniques in Head and Neck Surgery.* New York: Elsevier, 2007; 18: 99–104.

21.   Westphal K, Maeser D, Scheifler G, Lischke V, Byhahn C. PercuTwist: a new single-dilator technique for percutaneous tracheostomy. *Anesth Analg* 2003; 96: 229–32.

22.   Frova G, Quintel M. A new simple method for percutaneous tracheostomy: controlled rotating dilation: a preliminary report. *Intensive Care Med* 2002; 28(3): 299–303.

23.   Kumar M, Jaffery A, Jones M. Short term complications of percutaneous tracheostomy: experience of a district general hospital-otolaryngology department. *J Laryngol Otol* 2002; 116: 1025–7.

24.   Steele AP, Evans HW, Afaq MA, *et al.* Long-term follow-up of Griggs percutaneous tracheostomy with spiral CT and questionnaire. *Chest* 2000; 117: 1430–3.

25.   Sviri S, Samie R, Roberts BL, *et al.* Long-term outcomes following percutaneous tracheostomy using the Griggs technique. *Anaesth Intensive Care* 2003; 31: 401–7.

26.   Dollner R, Verch M, Schweiger P, *et al.* Long-term outcome after Griggs tracheostomy. *J Otolaryngol* 2002; 31: 386–9.

27.   Higgins KM, Punthakee X. Meta-analysis comparison of open versus percutaneous tracheostomy. *Laryngoscope* 2007; 117(3): 447–54.

28.   Kluge S, Baumann H, Maier C, *et al.* Tracheostomy in the intensive care unit: a nationwide survey. *Anesth Analg* 2008; 107: 1639–43.

29.   Kost K. Percutaneous tracheostomy: a comparison of Ciaglia and Griggs techniques. *Crit Care* 2000; 4: 143–6.

30.   Paran H, Butnaru G, Hass I, *et al.* Evaluation of a modified percutaneous tracheostomy technique without bronchoscopic guidance. *Chest* 2004; 126: 868–81.

31.   Arola MK. Tracheostomy and its complications. A retrospective study of 794 tracheostomized patients. *Ann Chir Gynaecol* 1981; 70: 96–106.

32.   Cheng E, Fee W. Dilational versus standard tracheostomy: a meta-analysis. *Ann Otol Rhinol Laryngol* 2000; 109: 803–7.

Emergency surgical airways

Leonard Pott and Scott Goldstein

Case presentation

A 56-year-old obese man arrived in the emergency department with impending respiratory arrest. He appears apneic and is cyanotic. The patient was found in a park struggling to breathe and unable to speak. No medical history is available. The team is attempting to ventilate him with a bag-valve mask, with no apparent change in oxygenation. Three different senior staff physicians have attempted to intubate his trachea, without success. The on-call anesthetist is paged to assist with the patient's care. On arrival, the anesthesiologist uses a laryngoscope with a MAC 4 blade, finding her view of the hypopharynx is obscured by edema and blood with no view of the cords, even with repositioning or cricoid pressure. The patient is in critical need of an airway as he continues to deteriorate. The pulse-oximeter reading has dropped to 40% and the heart rate decreased from 120 to 50 beats per minute.

Introduction

The above case demonstrates the dire situation of "can't ventilate, can't intubate" (CVCI) in a patient who cannot breathe. CVCI is rare, but is a life-threatening situation that requires immediate surgical airway access, usually an emergent cricothyroidotomy. Both civilian and military providers are often required to manage the airway under severely compromised circumstances and with limited equipment [1]. In these situations, a cricothyroidotomy may be life saving. The frequency with which cricothyroidotomy is used differs between different providers and settings. Cricothyroidotomy may be necessary for up to 2.8% of all intubation attempts in an emergency department for trauma patients, whereas prehospital cricothyroidotomy by paramedics varies between 2.4% and 14% of all intubation attempts [2].

There have been great strides in the development of airway adjuncts used to avoid the need for emergent surgical airway, which range from laryngeal mask airways (LMA) and other supraglottic devices to video laryngoscopes such as the Glide-Scope (Verathon Medical, Bothell, WA, USA). However, each of these has its own limitations, in particular, expense, lack of availability, and lack of operator familiarity with the equipment. Although adjuncts are frequently helpful, success cannot be guaranteed with any airway device. A surgical airway remains the definitive intervention when intubation is difficult or impossible [3].

Tracheotomy Management: A Multidisciplinary Approach, ed. Peggy A. Seidman, David Goldenberg and Elizabeth H. Sinz. Published by Cambridge University Press.
© Cambridge University Press 2011.

History

Cricothyroidotomy or cricothyrotomy has been used throughout time. There is literature, albeit vague, that it was accomplished by the Greeks in about 100 BC, and then in the 1500s by Antonius Bracivalla and the 1800s by Trousseau for severe diphtheria [4]. In the 1930s, Dr. Chevalier Jackson of Pittsburgh Hospital described a "high tracheotomy" pointing out the benefit of opening the trachea, especially in children, when there is no other way to get air into the bronchioles [5]. In his paper, he calls this procedure the "last hope" and compares the morbidity and mortality to incising a superficial abscess. Dr. Jackson described his procedure in two steps: the first to split the skin from the thyroid cartilage to the sternum, and the second for the operator's finger to palpate and penetrate the trachea. He recommended waiting until ventilation is started to obtain hemostasis.

Cricothyroidotomy came back into favor after being used by Brantigan and Grow [7]. This paper rejuvenated the life-saving procedure known as the cricothyroidotomy. Since its publication, the use of cricothyroidotomy has been used in emergent situations with good success and lower complication rates than first feared.

Anatomy

An understanding of the visualized and palpable structures of the anterior neck and surrounding structures is important for success with this procedure. From caudal to cephalad they are the tracheal rings, cricoid cartilage, cricothyroid membrane, thyroid cartilage (the Adam's apple), thyrohyoid membrane, hyoid bone, submandibular space, and mandible (Figure 4.1). While these features are always present, they may not always be easily palpated and identified due to anatomical differences, obesity, trauma, swelling, or scarring. The most important features to identify by palpation are the cricoid cartilage and thyroid cartilage to locate the cricothyroid membrane [8].

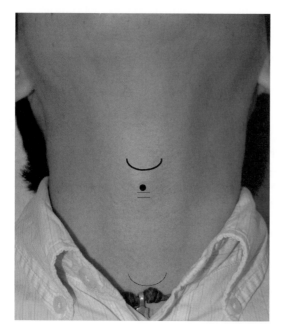

Figure 4.1 External anatomy landmarks:
Upper curved line: thyroid notch
Filled circle: cricothyroid membrane
Double straight line: cricoid cartilage
Lower curved line: sternal notch

The cricothyroid membrane is composed of fibroelastic tissue bordered by the cricothyroid muscles laterally, thyroid cartilage superiorly, and cricoid ring inferiorly. The width of the membrane is usually less than 2–3 cm in the horizontal plane, and averages about 8 mm at the midline in the vertical plane [8]. The vocal cords lie above the incision site and are protected by the thyroid cartilage, so cord injury should be avoidable.

Indications

- Patients requiring airway management that cannot be intubated by the oral or nasal route.
- Known or likely unstable cervical spine where manipulation of the neck is contraindicated.
- Severe maxillofacial trauma.
- Edema of the glottis and inability to visualize the vocal cords.
- Severe oropharyngeal or tracheobronchial hemorrhage.
- Fracture of the base of the skull.
- Foreign body obstruction of airways.

Contraindications [8]

- A less invasive method is possible to secure a patent airway (e.g., intubation).
- Patients under 5 years of age. (Although a needle cricothyroidotomy may be done, a formal tracheotomy is preferred.)
- Fracture of the larynx.
- Transection of the trachea with retraction of the distal end into the mediastinum.
- Laryngeal pathology.

Classification of cricothyroidotomy techniques

The ideal technique should provide for oxygenation and ventilation, be quick, easy to learn and perform, and be readily available [9–11]. A wide variety of kits are now commercially available to establish a cricothyroidotomy using different approaches. These techniques can be classified based on features they have in common. The fundamental difference between techniques is how the procedure is approached and how the airway lumen is entered: either by needle puncture or blade incision [11].

Needle puncture techniques

Needle puncture techniques are based on equipment originally developed for vascular access. Two different approaches exist:

(1) A needle puncture is performed to access the tracheal lumen and then a cannula can be passed over the needle.

(2) A needle is placed and a wire passed through the needle (Seldinger technique). In the Seldinger technique, the wire is then used as a guide for subsequent dilator and tube placement. The dilator can be used to ventilate before the definitive cricothyroidotomy cannula is placed.

Technique: needle cricothyroidotomy

1. Place the patient supine with the neck in either neutral or extended position.

2. Assemble the (usually 12 or 14 gauge) over-the-needle catheter attached to a 5-ml syringe. Some advocate putting saline in the syringe to make air bubbles more obvious.

3. Prep the neck using antiseptic solution.

4. Identify the cricothyroid membrane between the cricoid cartilage and the thyroid cartilage.

5. Stabilize the trachea with the thumb and forefinger of one hand to prevent lateral movement of the airway during the procedure.

6. Puncture the skin in the midline with the needle attached to the syringe, directly over the cricothyroid membrane. Recommended angle varies from 90 degrees with the neck to 45 degrees directed inferiorly. A small incision with a scalpel may facilitate passage of the needle through the skin.

7. While applying negative pressure to the syringe, carefully advance the needle through the cricothyroid membrane. Aspiration of air signifies entry into the tracheal lumen.

8. Redirect the needle inferiorly (caudad) and advance slightly, being careful not to perforate the posterior wall of the trachea.

9. Remove the syringe and withdraw the needle while advancing the catheter downward into position. Reassess the position of the catheter within the trachea by verifying air return into the syringe attached to the catheter.

10. Attach the oxygen tubing over the catheter needle hub to provide jet ventilation.

11. Observe chest rise to confirm ventilation and determine duration of insufflation.

12. One individual must do nothing except maintain the cannula stability.

The equipment to perform this procedure can be purchased in kits or taken from routinely available medical supplies. Each kit comes with specific instructions and these should ideally be reviewed by personnel who might be required to perform this procedure.

Once access to the trachea has been established via the cricothyroid membrane using a needle technique, the patient needs to be oxygenated and ventilated. The diameter of the lumen cannula will determine the resistance to gas flow and, therefore, size of the tidal volume that can be delivered for a given driving pressure and a given inspiratory time. A high-pressure system can be used to ventilate and/or oxygenate the patient. Low-pressure systems are based on bag-mask ventilation and, typically, use oxygen at pressures under 3 psi (0.2 atm, 150 mmHg). High-pressure oxygen is obtained from wall oxygen outlets, typically at approximately 50 psi (3.3 atm, 2600 mmHg). Low-pressure systems can be used to prevent hypoxemia, but can rapidly fail at ventilation (within 60 s) [2].

Jet ventilators

High-pressure oxygen requires a specialized system to deliver controlled volumes and because of the high pressures involved, these systems are commonly called "jet ventilators." Commercial products are available to provide controlled high-pressure oxygen, such as the Saunders injector or the Manujet (VBM Medizintechnik GmbH, Sulz, Germany). The equipment consists of low-compliance tubing to deliver and contain the high pressure, some form of valve that allows the operator to control the duration of the high-pressure gas stream, low-compliance tubing to connect to the cricothyroidotomy cannula, which includes an appropriate connection (usually a Luer lock), and ideally a mechanism to regulate the pressure.

Before attaching the jet ventilator to the patient, the equipment must be checked. The steps involved in using the equipment include:

(1) Attach the tubing to the high-pressure oxygen outlet (30–50 psi).

(2) Hold the patient end of the tubing firmly before opening the valve (pulling the valve trigger). This is very important because the high pressure may cause the tip to swing wildly, which may result in significant injury to persons or damage to equipment.

(3) Use the pressure regulator to decrease to the lowest pressure likely to provide satisfactory flow through the cannula to ensure adequate ventilation.

(4) Attach equipment to the patient's cannula.

(5) Apply short (0.5–1 s) bursts of high-pressure oxygen.

(6) Ensure adequate chest movement by inspection. It is not generally possible to measure the delivered volume.

(7) Ensure adequate escape of gas to prevent overinflation of the chest. Watch the degree of chest rise and fall at all times.

Significant risks are associated with jet ventilation, which include:

(1) Barotrauma to the lung, due to excessive inflation pressure.

(2) Pneumothorax and tension pneumothorax.

(3) Subcutaneous emphysema.

Jet ventilation is typically used when the cannula lumen is narrow, which means that adequate exhalation via the cannula is unlikely. The insufflated volume usually escapes past the surgical airway to the glottis and through the upper airway. In the case of complete upper airway obstruction to both inspiration and expiration, no gas escapes, the chest does not deflate, and intrathoracic pressure will rise, which may lead to the development of a tension pneumothorax. If the escape of inflated gas cannot be confirmed, jet ventilation must be stopped immediately. Another reason why inflated gas may not escape is that the gas has been injected into subcutaneous tissue rather than into the bronchial tree. This can be a rapidly lethal complication and the jet ventilation must be stopped immediately. The development of subcutaneous emphysema makes subsequent surgical airway access exceptionally difficult.

Blade incision techniques

With blade incision techniques (surgical cricothyroidotomy), the operator uses a surgical scalpel blade to incise the skin and then open the cricothyroid membrane in a horizontal direction to produce a hole through which a tube is placed. The difference between surgical techniques is how the aperture in the cricothyroid membrane is maintained before tube insertion. This step is important because if the opening moves it may be difficult to reidentify it, especially if there is bleeding.

(1) The classical description uses a tracheal hook to fix the cricoid cartilage and a Trousseau dilator to extend the opening.

(2) The four-step technique uses the scalpel handle both to control the opening and to aid in dilation.

(3) The three-step technique inserts a bougie to control the opening and to serve as a guide for tube placement.

Technique: blade incision cricothyroidotomy
Surgical cricothyroidotomy

1. Place the patient supine with the neck in a neutral or extended position.

2. Obtain the needed equipment.

3. Prep the neck using antiseptic solution and anesthetize the area, if there is time.

4. Identify by palpation the thyroid notch, cricothyroid membrane, the sternal notch, and hyoid bone for orientation.

5. Stabilize the thyroid with the non-dominant hand, keeping the skin taut over the thyroid notch. This is important in order not to lose the anatomical landmarks during the procedure.

6. Make a *vertical* skin incision (~2cm) over the cricothyroid membrane. Locate the membrane and then carefully incise *horizontally* (McGill et al., 1982) (1.5cm) through the lower half of the membrane. If available, a tracheal hook can be used to stabilize the larynx especially in the patient with a fat neck or hypermobile larynx.

7. Insert the scalpel handle into the incision and rotate it 90 degrees to open the airway. Extend the incision laterally for approximately 1 cm on each side of the midline.

8. Insert an appropriately sized, cuffed endotracheal tube or tracheotomy tube into the cricothyroid membrane incision, directing the tube distally into the trachea. The tube should always be aimed caudad.

9. Inflate the cuff and ventilate the patient using capnography to confirm ventilation.

10. Observe bilateral lung inflation and auscultate the chest to assure placement in trachea.

11. Secure the endotracheal tube to the patient.

Rapid four-step technique

Brofeldt, BT, Panacek, EA, Richards, JR. An Easy Cricothyrotomy Approach: The Rapid Four-Step Technique. *Acad Emer Med* 1996; 3:1060–1063.

1. **Palpation:** Palpate the cricothyroid membrane with the index finger of the nondominant hand. The middle finger and thumb palpate the carotid pulses and stabilize the trachea.

2. **Incision:** With the dominant hand, make a horizontal incision over the skin. Make a subsequent horizontal incision into the inferior aspect of the cricothyroid membrane. Push the scalpel through the membrane, creating a 2.5 cm horizontal incision. This eliminates the need for an extension of the incision or spreading the incision transversely as is usually recommended.

3. **Traction:** With the nondomianant hand, place the tracheal hook at the superior margin of the cricoid ring and apply caudal traction with the nondominant hand resting on the patient's sternum.

4. **Intubation:** Insert the tube into the trachea with the dominant hand. Remove the tracheal hook and inflate the cuff.

Rapid three-step technique (Figure 4.2) [12]

1. **Skin incision:** Cleanse the neck. Grasp the larynx with the nondominant hand, using the index finger to identify the thyroid cartilage, cricithyroid membrane, and cricoids ring. Using the dominant hand, make a vertical incision over the cricothyroid membrane. Palpate the cricothyroid membrane with the nondominant index finger through the incision.

2. **Incision of the cricothyroid membrane:** Move the nondominant index finger and make a 5 mm horizontal incision through the cricothyroid membrane. Place an elastic bougie through the hole into the trachea, and advance until resistance is appreciated, indicating impact with the carina or right mainstem bronchus.

3. **Endotracheal tube placement:** Using the bougie as a stylet, advance the endotracheal tube up to the cricothyroid membrane. Align the bevel of the endotracheal tube with the horizontal incision into the the cricothyroid membrane and apply gentle pressure to advance the endotracheal tube into the trachea until the cuff has just disappeared. Remove the bougie and inflate the cuff.

Complications

The rate and nature of the complications associated with a cricothyroidotomy depend on the choice of technique, skill level of the operator, and patient factors. Overall, a serious complication rate of 15–20% is considered representative [2,9,10,14].

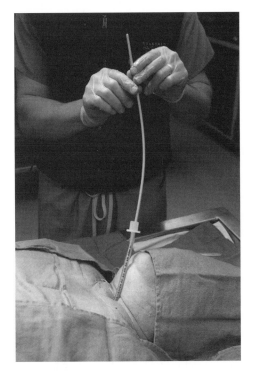

Figure 4.2 Emergency surgical airway: Three-step or Bougie technique. Copyright Darren Braude.

Complications include:

- Obstruction or kinking of the cannula.
- Anatomical misplacement of the device, which will lead to a failure to oxygenate/ventilate.
- Bleeding.
- Damage to adjacent structures such as the esophagus, posterior trachea, or laryngeal cartilages.
- Hypercapnia.
- Subcutaneous emphysema.
- Barotrauma.
- Pneumothorax.

Because needle cannulation limits the ability to ventilate patients, it is frequently converted to a surgical airway [1]. Surgical cricothyroidotomy is also inadequate for long-term ventilation and is frequently converted to a formal tracheotomy.

Recommendations

Because of logistic issues involved with supplying the necessary equipment throughout the institution, and with providing effective training to all relevant staff, it is not feasible to have practitioners using a large variety of different techniques. It is important that an agreement be reached by all stakeholders to use one technique. Important considerations are:

(1) *Speed of insertion.* As a cricothyroidotomy is a rescue procedure, which will be used once it has been established that oral or nasal intubation is impossible, and frequently once the patient is already hypoxic, it is essential that the procedure be performed rapidly. Studies examining how quickly the cricothyroidotomy airway can be established often do not include the preparation time, and have varying results. It has also been shown that personnel often do not know where the difficult airway equipment is found [15], favoring the choice of technique that uses common medical equipment such as a scalpel and endotracheal tube. In these situations, the degree of complexity of the equipment becomes an important consideration. It has been shown that the time to prepare a jet ventilation system may be excessively long, so the choice of technique will favor an approach that will allow for bag-valve ventilation. Studies comparing techniques are frequently done using inexperienced, and often untrained, subjects. Nonetheless, we suggest that all personnel who may potentially be called upon to perform a cricothyroidotomy must be adequately trained on some form of simulator (see below) with periodic refresher training [9,10,13,16,17]. Due to the emergency nature of this procedure, the most experienced person immediately available, regardless of discipline, should perform the procedure.

(2) *Situation.* A cricothyroidotomy may be performed in the pre-hospital or hospital setting. In the pre-hospital environment, it is very unusual to have high-pressure oxygen, and a recent review by Scrase and Woollard concluded there is no place for needle cricothyroidotomy with low-pressure ventilation systems in adult patients in the pre-hospital setting [2].

(3) *Risk of trauma.* Needle cannulation, because of the smaller diameter cannulae, and avoidance of an incision in a potentially vascular region, has the advantage of causing less trauma. Bleeding, which may obscure vision and access, is by far the most significant complication of the surgical approach. However, needle cannulation techniques often require the use of jet ventilation, which may be unavailable and may be associated with an increased risk of severe pulmonary trauma.

(4) *Efficacy of ventilation [13].* Exhalation is passive and requires a low resistance pathway. In the presence of complete supraglottic obstruction a cannula with a large lumen must be used to allow the escape of expired gas. While some needle and dilation techniques allow the passage of a large cannula, these procedures are time-consuming. On the other hand, incomplete upper airway obstruction prevents adequate ventilation because gas escapes proximally, particularly with poor pulmonary compliance. This necessitates the use of cuffed tubes [13]. The surgical approach will likely provide better ventilation.

(5) *Experience.* Anesthesiologists have much experience with using catheter and needle puncture techniques for vascular access while surgeons are extremely comfortable with a blade. This experience may influence the choice of technique but may be altered by appropriate training [18,19].

(6) *Cost.* If a kit (e.g., the Melker, Quicktrach, Patil) is chosen, then it is essential that these kits are available at all locations where they may be required. Because this may involve many sites, the total cost of the equipment may be high. In addition, regular simulator practice is necessary, which will also consume equipment resources and add to the total cost. Surgical techniques involve readily available equipment such as a scalpel and endotracheal tube, which are also low cost, giving surgical techniques a distinct advantage.

Post-cricothyroidotomy management

(1) *Assess the adequacy of oxygenation.* If the patient is still poorly oxygenated, determine the need for another approach. Needle cannulation is seldom sufficient to maintain oxygenation and ventilation for long, so this technique is frequently converted to formal tracheotomy [1].

(2) *Assess the continuing need for a cricothyroidotomy.* In a number of cases, the initial problem will have resolved and the device can be removed. This is best done in a controlled environment where facilities exist for airway support in case of bleeding, swelling, or reoccurrence of the initial pathology. If the airway remains compromised, for example in the case of severe facial trauma or facial burns, an otolaryngology consultation is recommended with a view to performing a formal tracheotomy.

Cricothyroidotomy training

Simulation is an important component of training and instruction in airway management, especially cricothyroidotomy because it is seldom performed. Without practice, the rate of successful placement is low. Practice on animals is expensive and can be problematic socially, and practice on living human patients is unethical and impractical. The various simulators used each have their own advantages and disadvantages; however, this practice is invaluable for skills' practice [9,11,19–23].

Mannequins

Plastic mannequins are commercially available, and various investigators have constructed cheap and simple cricothyroidotomy simulators from household materials. They allow the learner to practice the sequence of steps involved in the procedure, but are associated with major disadvantages. The mannequin's "tissue" consists of artificially clear layers, does not bleed, and does not retract. These limitations are felt to discriminate positively towards large bore cannulae and surgical techniques, and affect the validity of cricothyroidotomy research studies [10,11,16,24].

Animal preparations

Both live and dead animal preparations have been used. If live animals are used then it is important to ensure their welfare. The type of animal is chosen to mimic human anatomy as much as possible, so sheep, dogs, and pigs are frequently used [19,25,26].

Cadavers

The use of recently dead cadavers is the most realistic simulator but logistic considerations limit the availability of this model for routine instruction and assessment [9,17].

Significant controversy exists about which model is best. As correlation studies using living human subjects are impossible, the answer will not be established with certainty. The problem for research studies is that various forms of simulator are not considered equivalent to each other. However, no matter what type of simulator is used, it is important that the training be comprehensive and involves some form of competency assessment, and that regular refresher training is provided. However, the optimal method, intensity, and frequency of this training have yet to be determined [19,22]. Wong et al., using a mannequin model, found that success rate plateaued at five attempts [10,11,17,19,22,23].

All emergency airway providers, anesthesiologists, emergency medicine physicians, surgeons, emergency medical technicians, and military medical personnel should be completely familiar with at least one effective technique to provide an emergency cricothyroidotomy.

Conclusions

The case at the beginning of this chapter was managed by rapidly performing an emergency cricothyroidotomy. Using the three-step technique, an incision is made through the skin and cricoid membrane, an Eschmann bougie was introduced into the trachea, and a size 6.0 cuffed endotracheal tube inserted into the trachea [12]. The patient was immediately ventilated using a bag-ventilator (Ambu) with 100% oxygen. Once the patient was reoxygenated and stabilized, he was referred to surgery for airway assessment.

Depending on the patient's condition, a decision will need to be made whether to convert the cricothyroidotomy to a tracheotomy, to remove the cricothyroidotomy tube and insert an oral or nasal endotracheal tube, or to simply remove the tube and allow the patient to maintain his own airway.

References

1. Price RJ, Laird C. A survey of surgical airway experiences and equipment among immediate care doctors. *Emerg Med J* 2009; **26**: 438–41.

2. Scrase I, Woollard M. Needle vs surgical cricothyroidotomy: a short cut to effective ventilation. *Anaesthesia* 2006; **61**: 962–74.

3. Johansen K, Holm-Knudsen RJ, Charabi B, Kristensen MS, Rasmussen LS. Cannot ventilate – cannot intubate an infant: surgical tracheostomy or transtracheal cannula? *Pediatr Anesthesia* 2010; **20**: 987–93.

4. Parrillo JE, Dellinger RP. Critical care medicine: principles of diagnosis and management of the adult. 225.

5. Jackson C. Tracheotomy. *Laryngoscope* 1909; **19**: 285–90.

6. Jackson C. High tracheotomy and other errors the chief cause of chronic laryngeal stenosis. *Surg Gynecol Obstet* 1921; **32**: 392.

7. Brantigan CO, Grow JB Sr. Cricothyroidotomy: elective use in respiratory problems requiring tracheotomy. *J Thorac Cardiovasc Surg* 1976; **71**: 72–81.

8. Boon JM, Abrahams PH, Meiring JH, Welch T. Cricothyroidotomy; a clinical anatomy review. *Clin Anat* 2004; **17**(6): 478–86.

9. Eisenburger P, Laczika K, List M, *et al.* Comparison of convential surgical versus Seldinger technique emergency cricothyroidotomy performed by inexperienced clinicians. *Anesthesiology* 2000; **92**: 687–90.

10. Vadodaria BS, Gandi SD, McIndoe AK. Comparison of four different emergency airway access equipment sets on a human patient simulator. *Anaesthesia* 2004; **59**: 73–9.

11. Dimitriadis JC, Paoloni R. Emergency cricothyroidotomy: a randomised crossover study of four methods. *Anaesthesia* 2008; **63**: 1204–8.

12. MacIntyre A, Markarian MK, Carrison D, *et al.* Three-step emergency cricothyroidotomy. *Military Med* 2007; **12**: 1228–30.

13. Sulaiman L, Tighe SQM, Nelson RA. Surgical vs wire-guided cricothyroidotomy: a randomized crossover study of cuffed and uncuffed tracheal tube insertion. *Anaesthesia* 2006; **61**: 565–70.

14. Fikkers BG, van Vught S, van der Hoeven JG, van den Hoogen FJA, Marres HAM. Emergency cricothyrotomy: a randomised crossover trial comparing the wire-guided and catheter-over-needle techniques. *Anaesthesia* 2004; **59**: 1008–11.

15. Green L. Can't intubate, can't ventilate! A survey of knowledge and skills in a large teaching hospital. *Eur J Anaesth* 2009; **26**: 480–3.

16. Lacquiere A, Heard AMB. Emergency cricothyroidotomy: training is paramount and oxygenation is the aim. *Anaesthesia* 2009; **64**: 447–8.

17. Schaumann N, Lorenz V, Schellongowski P, *et al.* Evaluation of Seldinger technique emergency cricothyroidotomy versus standard surgical cricothyroidotomy in 200 cadavers. *Anesthesiology* 2005; **102**: 7–11.

18. Wong DT, Lai K, Chung FF, Ho RY. Cannot intubate-cannot ventilate and difficult intubation strategies: results of a Canadian national survey. *Anesth Analg* 2005; **100**: 1439–46.

19. Heard AMB, Green RJ, Eakins P. The formulation and introduction of a "can't intubate, can't ventilate" algorithm into clinical practice. *Anaesthesia* 2009; **64**: 601–8.

20. Rosenstock C, Hansen EG, Kristensen MS, *et al.* Qualitative analysis of unanticipated difficult airway management. *Acta Anaesthesiol Scand* 2006; **50**: 290–7.

21. Chang RS, Hamilton RJ, Carter WA. Declining rate of cricothyroidotomy in trauma patients with an emergency medicine residency: implication for skills training. *Acad Emerg Med* 1998; **5**: 247–51.

22. Wong DT, Prabhu AJ, Coloma M, Imasogie N, Chung FF. What is the minimum training required for successful cricothyroidotomy? *Anesthesiology* 2003; **98**: 349–53.

23. Kulkarni NV. Cricothyrodotomy pig model flawed. *Emerg Med J* 2009; **26**: 623.

24. Varaday SS, Yentis SM, Clarke S. A homemade model for training in cricothyroidotomy. *Anaesthesia* 2004; **59**: 1012–15.

25. Paladino L, DuCanto J, Manoach S. Development of a rapid, safe, fiber-optic guided, single-incision cricothyroidotomy using a large ovine model: a pilot study. *Resuscitation* 2009; **80**: 1066–9.

26. Ward KR, Menegazzi JJ, Yealy DM, *et al.* Translaryngeal jet ventilation and end-tidal PCO_2 monitoring during varying degrees of upper airway obstruction. *Ann Emerg Med* 1991; **20**: 1193–7.

Chapter 5

Congenital, embryological, and anatomic variations, and their association with pediatric tracheotomy

Elliot Regenbogen

Case presentation

Our patient was born at 37 weeks via cesarian section to a 31-year-old woman who was group B Streptococcus and rapid plasma reagin positive. The child's Apgar scores were 7 and 8, she weighed 3.3 kg, and had dysmorphic features. She was intubated with difficulty soon after birth for respiratory distress. On examination, the child had a dysmorphic facies and a diagnosis of Pierre–Robin syndrome was made.

Embryology

At 24–36 days of gestation, the tracheobronchial tree develops initially from a bulge at the laryngotracheal groove on the ventral wall of the pharynx. Endoderm gives rise to the epithelium of the trachea, bronchi, and alveoli. Mesoderm gives rise to the muscle, cartilage, and connective tissue. By the 28th day, the right and left lung buds have formed and as the lung buds elongate, lateral invagination of mesoderm forms the separation of the esophagus and trachea. Cartilage appears in the trachea at 10 weeks. Defective or incomplete separation by the tracheoesophageal septum is one of the most frequent congenital anomalies producing tracheoesophageal fistula (TEF). As laryngeal and bronchial development is a separate process, malformations such as tracheal stenosis may occur in the face of a normal larynx and bronchial tree [2].

Anatomic variations

Anatomic variations that can influence the planning and success of a tracheotomy may be broadly grouped into extrinsic and intrinsic causes.

Extrinsic airway obstruction

Congenital lesions

Nasal obstruction

During the first 6 weeks of life, children are obligate nasal breathers. Apnea will result unless the mouth is opened if bilateral nasal obstruction is present, depending on the degree of

Tracheotomy Management: A Multidisciplinary Approach, ed. Peggy A. Seidman,
David Goldenberg and Elizabeth H. Sinz. Published by Cambridge University Press.
© Cambridge University Press 2011.

Table 5.1

Extrinsic airway obstruction	Intrinsic airway obstruction
Congenital	**Congenital**
Nasal Obstruction	Tracheal agenesis/atresia
Pyriform aperture stenosis	Tracheal stenosis
Choanal atresia	Complete tracheal rings
Oropharynx	Tracheal webs
Retrognathia/tracheobronchomalacia	Tracheomalacia
	Laryngomalacia
Vascular	Vocal Cord Paralysis
Arterial/venous/lymphatic/mixed	Laryngeal Webs
Bronchogenic Cysts	Laryngeal Clefts
Esophageal Anomalies	80% tracheomalacia
Atresia	20% TEF
Tracheoesophageal fistula (TEF)	Subglottic Hemangiomas
Inflammatory/Infectious	Congenital High Airway Obstruction Syndrome (CHAOS)
Lymphadenopathy	Craniofacial Syndromes
– neck	**Inflammatory/Infectious**
– mediastinum	Croup
Deep Space Infection	Tracheitis
Esophageal Foreign Bodies	Relapsing Polychondritis
Neoplasm	**Metabolic**
Lymphoma	Hunter syndrome
Rhabdomyosarcoma	**Trauma**
Neurogenic tumors	**Primary tracheal neoplasm**
Germ cell tumors	Squamous Cell Carcinoma
Metastasis	Adenoid Cystic Carcinoma
Thyroid	Hemangioma
	Papillomatosis

obstruction. Unilateral obstruction may go undiagnosed for years, presenting only as unilateral rhinorrhea and obstruction.

The etiology of the obstruction may include an anterior congenital nasal pyriform aperture stenosis (which is rare), a tumor, or choanal atresia. Choanal atresia may be unilateral or bilateral and may be associated with congenital anomalies, in particular CHARGE syndrome (coloboma, heart defects, genitourinary disorders, and ear abnormalities). Those with CHARGE may have more severe nasal obstruction at birth as well as malacia of the pharynx, hypopharynx, and larynx. If this is the case, tracheotomy will be required during initial management.

Oropharynx

Obstructing retrognathia usually will cause problems during the neonatal period. However, obstruction may become a problem during later development such as at the time of an incidental surgical procedure or with the development of sleep apnea. Tracheotomy is considered for those with persistent airway obstruction and feeding difficulties. As tracheo-bronchomalacia may be associated with retrognathia, one must be aware that tracheotomy may not alleviate all symptoms of obstruction.

Vascular anomalies

Vascular malformations may be venous, lymphatic, or mixed venolymphatic. Although these lesions are often soft and compressible, giant malformations of the neck and/or chest can compromise the airway by mass effect [3].

Vascular malformations resulting from abnormal development of the aorta and its branches can result in tracheal and esophageal compression or displacement. The most common type of vascular ring is a double aortic arch or right aortic arch with an aberrant left subclavian artery and patent ductus arteriosus. Symptoms that may be associated with vascular rings include wheezing, stridor, feeding difficulties, choking episodes, or aspiration pneumonia. Tracheotomy may be necessary to provide preoperative relief of the obstruction, albeit with the risk of tracheal erosion into the compressing vascular structure, or post-operatively to stent a segment of tracheomalacia.

Bronchogenic cysts

Bronchogenic cysts that form from abnormal budding of the foregut are some of the most common cystic lesions of the chest. While most occur at the carina, they may be present anywhere along the respiratory tract.

Esophageal anomalies

The most common congenital malformation of the esophagus is esophageal atresia, with or without TEF [2]. They are thought to be caused by an abnormality in the formation and division of the primitive foregut. The most common type of esophageal atresia has an associated distal TEF. Associated conditions include: trisomy 18, 21, and VATER/VACTERL anomalies (vertebral, anal, cardiac, TEF, esophageal atresia, renal, limb); a history of polyhydramnios, excess mouth secretions, respiratory distress, and inability to pass an esophageal catheter into the stomach. Air in the distal gastrointestinal tract suggests TEF. Tracheomalacia frequently accompanies this [3].

Infectious, inflammatory

Deep neck space infections can exert a direct mass affect causing tracheal narrowing, especially when the mediastinum or hilar lymphadenopathy is involved. Esophageal foreign bodies may present with symptoms of airway compromise or with deep neck infection due to perforation.

Neoplasm and goiter

While lymphoma is the most common childhood neoplasm that can compromise airways, other causes include infantile rhabdomyosarcoma, neurogenic tumors, and germ cell tumors. In adults, extrinsic airway neoplasms can include lymphoproliferative, metastatic, and primary tumor of any non-airway structure of the neck.

The extension of a thyroid goiter in the neck into the inferior thoracic inlet behind the sternum is known as a retrosternal or substernal goiter. The majority are extensions of the cervical thyroid gland but rarely an ectopic mass may be present. Most substernal goiters are in the anterior mediastinum but up to 10–15% may be posterior. In addition to cervical findings, clinical manifestations may include dyspnea, hoarseness, superior vena cava syndrome, and dysphagia [4].

Although tracheomalacia with substernal goiter is infrequent, when a substernal goiter has been present for more than 5 years with significant tracheal compression, the likelihood of tracheomalacia and tracheotomy are increased [5].

Intrinsic airway obstruction

Congenital

Tracheal agenesis/atresia

Payne first described tracheal agenesis in 1900 after a failed tracheotomy attempt on an infant. The incidence of tracheal agenesis, which is not usually compatible with life, is reportedly less than 1:50 000 with male predominance. This malformation has been divided into three types: type I (20%), tracheal atresia with short distal trachea, normal bronchi, and TEF; type II (60%), complete atresia but normal bifurcation and bronchi; and type III (20%), no trachea with bronchi arising from the esophagus [6].

Tracheal stenosis, and complete tracheal rings and webs

Congenital tracheal stenosis is narrowing of the trachea due to the presence of complete, as opposed to normal "C"-shaped, tracheal rings (Figure 5.1). This is a rare condition and life threatening. Half of those diagnosed with this condition will have an area of stenosis of 2 mm, which is smaller than the smallest endotracheal tube and standard tracheotomy tubes. Stenosis may occur focally or in segments, and rarely, as a complete cartilaginous sleeve. The alteration in diameter rather than length has a greater effect on resistance to airflow, as length varies resistance linearly while a change in diameter will affect resistance to the fourth power. Congenital tracheal stenosis may be associated with congenital heart disease, TEF, and skeletal abnormalities. Treatments include tracheoplasty, resection with reanastomosis and stenting [6].

Congenital tracheal webs are rare presenting with stridor, wheezing, and recurrent respiratory infections. There is no associated deformity of the tracheal wall and its presence may be documented on computed tomography (CT) or endoscopy. The web is not associated with deformity of the tracheal cartilage or wall, and CT demonstrates a web-like structure traversing and narrowing the tracheal lumen.

Tracheomalacia

Tracheomalacia is a softening of the tracheal wall resulting in collapse and obstruction. Primary tracheomalacia is congenital and may be associated with other developmental defects such as a vascular ring or TEF. Secondary tracheomalacia is caused by an event resulting in softening of previously normal tracheal cartilage such as prolonged intubation.

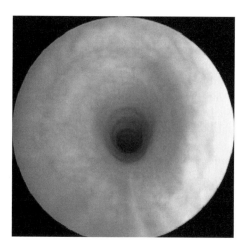

Figure 5.1 Complete tracheal rings from congenital tracheal anomalies.

Laryngomalacia

Laryngomalacia is the most common cause of stridor in the neonate. The stridor is worse during feeding, crying, and lying supine, and while it may worsen during the first 6 months of life in up to 50% of cases, almost all will resolve within 1 year. Approximately 5% will require surgical intervention due to severity of symptoms. While this may include tracheotomy, supraglottoplasty is preferred when possible [7].

Vocal cord paralysis

This is the second most common cause of stridor in newborns. It may be unilateral, bilateral, congenital, or iatrogenic. Almost all with bilateral paralysis will require tracheotomy.

Laryngeal webs

Incomplete recanalization of the glottic airway during embryogenesis results in a glottic web, which, depending on the degree of severity, may produce varied symptoms ranging from dysphonia, dyspnea, or true obstruction in laryngeal atresia. While associated congenital anomalies occur with a 10% frequency, there is a strong association between anterior glottic webs and velocardiofacial syndrome. Thick webs will require tracheotomy in approximately 40% of patients [7].

Laryngotracheal clefts

Congenital laryngeal clefts and laryngotracheal–esophageal clefts occur in approximately 1 of 2000 live births (Figure 5.2). Associated airway anomalies include tracheomalacia (80%) and TEF (20%) [7]. Clefting may be limited to the supraglottis or extend into the distal trachea and bronchi. Neonates present with a hoarse cry, the inability to handle secretions, cyanosis, choking, coughing, stridor, and recurrent pneumonia, depending on the length of the cleft. Before repair, the airway is often difficult to maintain. Often, tracheotomy is suggested; however, with some severe deformities, a tracheotomy may not secure the airway adequately. Custom-made, bifurcated, endotracheal and tracheotomy tubes have been described for maintaining these difficult airways with reasonable success [6].

Subglottic hemangiomas

These are associated with cutaneous hemangiomas more than 50% of the time. The natural history is one of a growth phase followed by spontaneous involution. Placement of a tracheotomy tube with planned decannulation between 1 and 2 years of age has been a traditional treatment plan. Resection or ablation of subglottic hemangiomas may be complicated by subsequent subglottic stenosis [7].

Congenital high airway obstruction syndrome and the ex utero intrapartum treatment procedure

Congenital high airway obstruction syndrome, severe complete obstruction of the fetal airway, may be suspected in fetal hydrops when ultrasound findings reveal enlarged echogenic lungs, flattened or inverted diaphragms, dilated airways, and mediastinal compression. Possible etiologies can include tracheal agenesis, atresia, or laryngotracheal cysts. The ex utero intrapartum treatment procedure may be performed to allow time to obtain an airway with tracheotomy while uteroplacental gas exchange is preserved via an intact umbilical cord.

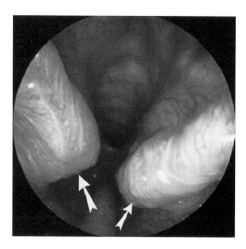

Figure 5.2 Preoperative endoscopic view of a type IIIb cleft.

Compared with cesarian section or vaginal delivery, the ex utero intrapartum treatment procedure, in congenital high airway obstruction syndrome, offers the potential for salvage and excellent long-term outcome [6].

Acquired

Inflammatory and infectious conditions

Croup, or laryngotracheobronchitis, is a common acute viral respiratory tract infection in children aged 6 months–3 years. Children typically present with signs of an upper respiratory illness, including a low-grade fever and barking cough. A frontal X-ray, including the neck, reveals hypopharyngeal overdistention and subglottic airway narrowing (a steeple sign). Bacterial tracheitis, which is considered life threatening, may present with similar symptoms but in general, the patient is more toxic and refractory to treatment. Radiography may demonstrate additional findings of tracheal membranes or tracheal wall irregularity.

Respiratory tract involvement may occur in up to half of patients with relapsing polychondritis. This rare condition involves recurrent inflammation of cartilaginous structures, including those of the larynx and trachea. Airway involvement is an indicator of poor prognosis and the leading cause of death. The CT finding of abnormalities sparing the posterior membranous wall is highly suggestive of relapsing polychondritis [3].

Metabolic conditions

Hunter syndrome is a rare genetic disorder primarily affecting males, in which there is an inability to break down certain mucopolysaccharides. The deposition of mucopolysaccharides in the walls of major airways results in progressive airway narrowing due to wall thickening and anteroposterior collapse [3].

Trauma

Direct trauma can result in cartilaginous damage and occlusion of the airway lumen by hemorrhage, edema, granulation tissue, scarring, or structural collapse. Pressure necrosis

Table 5.2 Craniofacial syndromes and associated airway anomalies [8]

Trachea	Larynx
Abnormal cartilage ring size or number	Atresia
1. Langer-type mesomelic dwarfism	1. Fraser syndrome
Bronchomalacia	2. Hypomandibular faciocranial
1. Apert syndrome	dysostosis
2. Ellis–van Creveld syndrome	3. 47 XXX syndrome
3. Fryn's syndrome	Laryngeal cleft
4. Hyperphalangism–facial anomaly–	1. G syndrome
hallus valgus–bronchomalacia	2. Pallister–Hall syndrome
5. Hypomandibular faciocranial dysostosis	Hypoplasia
6. Larsen's syndrome	1. Dysmorphic facies, omphalocele, spinal anomalies, learning
7. Pfeiffer's syndrome	disabilities and laryngeal hypoplasia
8. Pierre–Robin sequence	2. Fetal valproate syndrome
Cartilagenous tracheal sleeve	3. Marshall–Smith syndrome
1. Apert syndrome	4. Nager syndrome
2. Cloverleaf anomaly	5. Toriello–Carey syndrome
3. Crouzon's syndrome	Laryngeal web
4. Goldenhar's syndrome	1. Velocardiofacial syndrome
5. Pfeiffer syndrome	Laryngomalacia
6. Saethre–Chotzen syndrome	1. Apert syndrome
Net-like deformity	2. Freeman–Sheldon syndrome
1. Ellis–van Creveld syndrome	3. Larsen's syndrome
2. Fryn's syndrome	4. Marshall–Smith syndrome
Stenosis	5. Pfeiffer syndrome
1. Trisomy 21	6. Pierre–Robin syndrome
Tracheal cartilage plate defects	Stenosis
1. de la Chapelle dwarfism	1. Fraser syndrome
2. Rib–gap defect	2. Frontometaphyseal dysplasia
3. Treacher–Collins syndrome	3. Klippel–Feil syndrome
Tracheomalacia	4. Trisomy 21
1. Atelosteogenesis types 1 and 3	Vocal cord paralysis
2. Fetal valproate syndrome	1. Arthrogryposis multiplex congenita
3. Fryn's syndrome	2. Cri du chat
4. Kneist syndrome	3. Frontometaphyseal dysplasia
5. Hallerman–Streif syndrome	4. Klippel–Feil syndrome
6. Larsen's syndrome	
7. Metatropic dwarfism	

from intubation, with or without infection, can lead to malacia and/or fixed stenosis. Stenosis is usually at the level of the cricoid cartilage (the narrowest part of the upper airway and a solid ring), although when secondary to tracheotomy, placement will be lower.

Proliferative or neoplastic disease

Primary tracheal tumors are rare. In adults, 90% are malignant compared with only 10–30% in children. Squamous cell carcinoma and adenoid cystic carcinoma, in equal proportion, account for two-thirds of adult primary tracheal tumors [9].

The most common pediatric tracheobronchial tumors include hemangioma, bronchial carcinoid, and papillomatosis. Hemangiomas can be life threatening when subglottic, especially during the proliferative phase of the tumor. In this phase, there is a characteristic appearance on contrast CT and magnetic resonance [3].

Table 5.3 Classification of primary tracheal tumors [6]

Surface epithelium	Mesenchyme
Benign	*Benign*
Papilloma	Fibroma
Papillomatosis	Fibromatosis
Malignant	Benign fibrous histiocytoma
Squamous carcinoma in situ	Hemangioma
Squamous cell carcinoma	Hemangiopericytoma
Adenocarcinoma	Paraganglioma (chemodectoma)
Large cell undifferentiated carcinoma	Glomus tumor
Neuroendocrine tumors:	Leiomyoma
Typical and atypical carcinoids	Granular cell tumor
Large cell neuroendocrine tumor	Schwann cell tumors
Small cell carcinoma	Chondroma
Salivary glands	Chondroblastoma
Benign	*Malignant*
Pleiomorphic adenoma	Soft tissue type sarcomas
Mucus gland adenoma	Chondrosarcoma
Myoepithelioma	Malignant lymphomas
Oncocytoma	Other
Other	
Malignant	
Mucoepidermoid carcinoma	
Adenoid cystic carcinoma	
Carcinoma ex pleiomorphic adenoma	

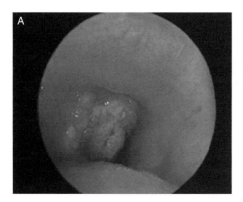 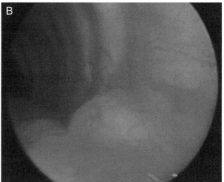

Figure 5.3 (A) Bronchoscopic view of a near-occlusive squamous cell tumour of the intrathoracic trachea. (B) Adenoid cystic tumor located at right cartilaginous pars membranacea groove.

In adults, tumors may not produce symptoms until a large portion of the tracheal lumen is occluded. Aside from dyspnea and wheezing, signs and symptoms may include hoarseness, dysphagia, hemoptysis, and stridor. Misdiagnosis such as asthma, chronic bronchitis, or chronic obstructive pulmonary disease is commonplace [9].

Conclusions

For the child presented at the beginning of this chapter, an elective tracheotomy was performed on day 11 of life after ruling out other congenital anomalies. The child did well with appropriate follow-up, meeting normal developmental milestones. She was evaluated at age 18m for revision of her tracheostoma and possible tracheal stenosis. The team felt that her mandibular growth was still insufficient and the trachea was widely patent, so they decided to reevaluate every 6 months. At age 36 months, growth was felt to be adequate and decannulation was planned.

References

1. Berrocal T, Madrid C, Novo S, *et al.* Congenital anomalies of the tracheobronchial tree, lung, and mediastinum: embryology, radiology, and pathology. *Radiographics* 2003; **24**: e17.

2. Yedururi S, Guillerman RP, Chung T, *et al.* Multimodality imaging of tracheobronchial disorders in children. *Radiographics* 2008; **28**(3): e29.

3. Xu J, Shen B, Li Y, *et al.* Enormous goiter in posterior mediastinum: report of 2 cases and literature review. *J Formos Med Assoc* 2009; **108**: 337–43.

4. White ML, Doherty GM, Gauger PG. Evidence-based surgical management of substernal goiter. *World J Surg* 2008; **32**: 1285–300.

5. Sandu K, Monnier P. Congenital tracheal anomalies. *Otolaryngol Clin North Am* 2007; **40**: 193–217.

6. Rutter MJ. Evaluation and management of upper airway disorders in children. *Semin Pediatr Surg* 2006; **15**: 116–23.

7. Papay FA, McCarthy VP, Eliachar I, Arnold J. Laryngotracheal anomalies in children with craniofacial syndromes. *J Craniofac Surg* 2002; **13**(2): 351–64.

8. Macchiarini P. Primary tracheal tumours. *Lancet Oncol* 2006; 7: 83–91.

Pediatric tracheotomy

Robert Yellon, Raymond Maguire, and Jay B. Tuchman

Case presentation

A two year-old girl with Down syndrome developed progressive stridor two weeks following routine endotracheal intubation for repair of atrioventricular septal defect. Stridor and airway obstruction progressed despite administration of helium-oxygen, corticosteroids and racemic epinephrine in the Intensive Care Unit. The child was rapidly transferred to the operating room where the anesthesiologist maintained bag mask ventilation and induced general anesthesia. The Otolaryngologist performed rigid bronchoscopy with a 3.0 bronchoscope and diagnosed a severe circumferential subglottic stenosis with a 2 mm lumen. Oxyhemoglobin desaturation occurred and the bronchoscope was passed through the stenosis, thereby securing the airway. An orderly tracheotomy was then successfully performed.

Introduction

The first known pediatric tracheotomy was performed in 1620 in Paris by Nicholas Habicot on a 16-year-old boy who swallowed a bag of coins, which subsequently became lodged in his esophagus and obstructed his airway. After performing the tracheotomy, the bag of coins was manipulated such that it would pass per rectum and the boy's life was preserved. Since the first pediatric tracheotomy, much has changed with regard to management of the pediatric airway. During the 1800s tracheotomy gained popularity in France where Armand Trousseau is credited for saving hundreds of children dying from diphtheria. Infectious diseases continued to be the predominant indication for tracheotomy until advances in neonatal medicine increased the survival of premature infants in the 1980s [1].

The development of advanced neonatal care and anesthesia techniques enabled patients to be intubated for prolonged periods leading to a rise in incidence of acquired subglottic stenosis and the survival of patients with ventilator-dependent respiratory failure. With this paradigm shift, indications for pediatric tracheotomy tube placement also changed from those of infectious etiology to that of respiratory support, airway obstruction, and pulmonary toilet for those with chronic aspiration (see Table 6.1).

The decision for tracheotomy tube placement should entail a detailed thought process and individualized plan for each patient. The increased burden of tracheotomy tube placement and required postoperative care may account for upwards of $900 000 in additional medical cost and prolonged hospitalization [3]. In addition to the increased economic cost, the mental

Tracheotomy Management: A Multidisciplinary Approach, ed. Peggy A. Seidman, David Goldenberg and Elizabeth H. Sinz. Published by Cambridge University Press.

Table 6.1 The current indications for pediatric tracheotomy placement [2]

Indications for pediatric tracheotomy
1. Airway obstruction (27%)
2. Neurologic deficit (25%)
3. Respiratory support (22%)
4. Trauma (17%)
5. Craniofacial syndromes (4%)

health burden weighs heavily on the family and increases with the severity of the child's illness. Family stress may manifest as increased rates of divorce or decreased quality of life for the caregiver, with less time and money for holidays or social activities [4].

Preoperative evaluation

When evaluating children for tracheotomy tube placement, it is important to communicate openly with anesthesia staff. Primary and secondary plans of securing the airway for tracheotomy should be prepared in advance. Attention to certain anatomical problems such as retrognathia, tongue base prolapse, macroglossia, or any glottic/supraglottic mass should be identified before the procedure. In addition, the child's medical history should be carefully reviewed, with specific attention paid to any previous intubations (difficult or not), laryngoscopy, bronchoscopy, and esophagoscopy. Flexible laryngoscopy is another useful means for evaluation of the airway, which may aid in the decision-making process.

When possible, it is preferable that tracheotomy be performed in the operating suite where adequate lighting, suction, equipment, and assistance are readily available. Access to multiple types and sizes of endotracheal and tracheotomy tubes, as well as, rigid bronchoscopy equipment is necessary. Securing the airway by artificial means before the child exhausts their respiratory reserve or progression to complete airway obstruction is paramount. This may be accomplished by direct laryngoscopy with intubation, rigid bronchoscopy, or flexible fiberoptic bronchoscopy with intubation. Multiple failed attempts at intubation may also precipitate acute obstruction from local edema in an already tenuous airway. Planned elective tracheotomy is always preferred over emergent bedside tracheotomy or cricothyroidotomy. In selected older children, awake tracheotomy under local anesthesia can be performed, especially in situations of laryngeal trauma where positive pressure ventilation may lead to subcutaneous emphysema or pneumothorax [5].

Anatomy

Knowledge of anatomical relationships is essential in performing any surgical procedure and the larynx is no exception. The neonatal and adult larynx differs in both form and position with implications for airway surgery (see Figures 6.1 and 6.2). The neonatal pharynx is vertically short with the tip of the epiglottis lying at the level of the first cervical vertebra (C1) and inferior margin of the cricoid at C4. This high epiglottic positioning and close approximation to the palate is thought to enable the infant to breathe and suckle simultaneously.

Mature   Infant

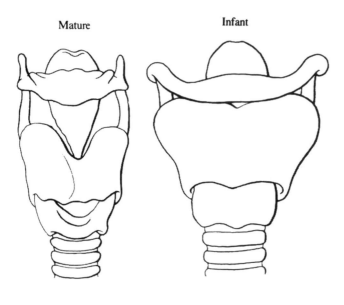

Figure 6.1 Anterior view comparing the adult and infant larynx. (From Bosma JF. *Anatomy of the Infant Head*. Baltimore: Johns Hopkins University Press, 1986, pp. 366–367.)

Mature   Infant

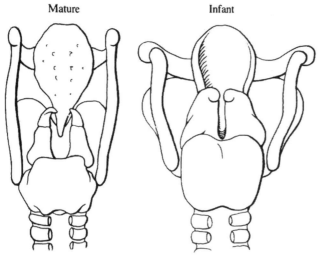

Figure 6.2 Posterior view comparing the adult and infant larynx. (From Bosma JF. *Anatomy of the Infant Head*. Baltimore: Johns Hopkins University Press, 1986, pp. 366–367.)

The laryngeal skeleton is also compact in the neonate with the thyroid cartilage telescoping vertically into the arch of the hyoid. The arytenoids are comparatively large secondary to a thick areolar submucosa. The dimensions of the neonatal glottis are 7 mm anteroposteriorly and 4 mm transversely. The narrowest part of the upper airway is the subglottis with a diameter of 4–5 mm [6].

As children continue to grow, the larynx descends in the neck with the cricoid lying at the level of C5 by age 2, C6 by age 5, and then at the adult position of between C6 and C7 at 15 years of age. Separation of the thyroid cartilage and hyoid bone also occurs throughout this process. Vocal fold length and proportion of the cartilaginous to membranous vocal fold also changes throughout childhood. Sixty to 75% of neonatal vocal fold length is comprised of cartilage from the vocal process of the arytenoid. The ratio of cartilaginous to membranous

Patient Age	Inner Diameter (mm)
Premature	
<1000 g	2.5
1000–2500 g	3.0
Neonate–6 months	3.0–3.5
6 months– 1 year	3.5–4.0
1–2 years	4.0–5.0
Beyond 2 years	$\dfrac{\text{Age in years} + 16}{4}$

Figure 6.3 Appropriate size endotracheal and tracheotomy tubes for infants and children. (From Cote CJ, Ryan JF, Todres ID, Goudsouzian NG. *A Practice of Anesthesia for Infants and Children*, 2nd edition. Philadelphia: WB Saunders, 1992.)

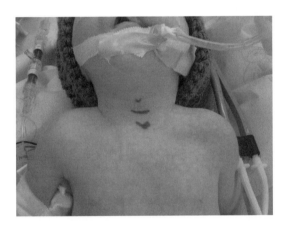

Figure 6.4 Surgical landmarks made before tracheotomy procedure outlining the sternal notch (inferior), incision (middle), and thyroid prominance (superior).

vocal fold is approximately 50:50 by 2 years of age with the membranous portion predominating after age 3.

The length of the neonatal trachea increases from 4 cm at birth to 12 cm in adulthood. The growth of the cartilaginous tracheal rings and annular ligaments accounts for the increased length until puberty. After puberty, the increased tracheal length is gained exclusively from the annular ligaments. Thus, closer approximation of the tracheal rings is found in children [6].

Technique

When performing a tracheotomy, the patient should be positioned on the operating table with the head flush to the end of the bed and a rolled towel placed under the shoulders to extend the neck. If necessary, the anesthesiologist may lift or tape the chin to provide maximal exposure. The anatomic landmarks of hyoid bone, thyroid notch, cricoid cartilage, and sternal notch are identified by palpation and an appropriate skin incision is marked (see Figure 6.4). All esophageal catheters should be removed as these may alter the anatomic relationships and provide a source of confusion of the esophagus for the trachea.

Local anesthetic is infiltrated into the marked site for a 1.5 cm horizontal skin incision. The skin incision should be located a minimum of one finger's breadth above the sternal notch but below the thyroid isthmus. This positioning allows the best exposure and least chance for a stretched and unsightly scar. Next, the skin is incised and underlying subcutaneous fat is removed thereby decreasing the distance from the skin to the trachea. The middle

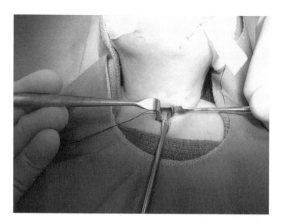

Figure 6.5 Tracheal rings are exposed and the right stay suture is placed. Two such sutures are placed in the paramedian position at the level of the 2nd and 3rd tracheal ring to secure the airway in cases of accidental decannulation in the immediate postoperative period.

layer of the deep cervical fascia should now be fully visible along with the strap muscles. The midline raphe of the sternohyoid muscles is identified, and using traction-counter traction principles, the strap muscles are divided vertically. This technique is repeated for the sternothyroid muscles and deeper connective tissue. The midline of the neck is relatively avascular and little bleeding is usually encountered. Deep dissection without adequate exposure is discouraged to avoid uncontrolled bleeding.

The strap muscles and connective tissue are pulled laterally with Senn retractors and the pretracheal fascia is visualized. Retraction must be performed with care as overzealous maneuvers may lead to vascular injuries or pneumothorax secondary to the high apical pleura in the pediatric patient. Next, the thyroid gland is either retracted superiorly or, if this is not possible, divided with electrocautery in infants or suture ligation in older children.

Nylon stay sutures are placed adjacent to the planned vertical tracheal incision (see Figure 6.5). Stay sutures will provide added security in case of accidental decannulation in the early postoperative period. The tracheotomy incision involves two to three tracheal rings usually between the second and fifth tracheal ring. Local anesthetic lie-lidocaine with epinephrine may be infiltrated into the planned vertical incision for hemostasis. Then, after alerting anesthesia staff, gentle traction is placed on the trachea using the stay sutures to pull anteriorly and laterally and the vertical tracheotomy incision is created. Secondary traction sutures are next placed on the right and left using 3–0 nylon. Care is taken to avoid crossing the stay sutures, which will later be marked with tape – "do not remove RIGHT and LEFT."

The endotracheal tube (ETT) is then withdrawn, such that the end of the tube lies just superior to the tracheal incision and an appropriate size tracheotomy tube is placed (see Figure 6.3). The tracheotomy tube should easily pass into the lumen of the trachea. Small or horizontal incisions allow unnecessary pressure on the tracheal ring superior to the tracheotomy tube possibly leading to suprastomal collapse. After the tracheotomy tube is placed the anesthesia circuit is connected and the ability to ventilate the patient adequately is assessed using capnography and chest rise. Twill tracheotomy ties are used to secure the tube around the patient's neck allowing for only one finger's breadth of space between the skin and the tie while the neck is flexed. Duoderm may be used as a barrier between the patient's skin and tracheotomy ties to prevent breakdown of the skin in the postoperative period.

The previously placed stay sutures are now taped to the patient's right and left chest, respectively, after they are tied loosely to prevent them from slipping out (see Figure 6.6).

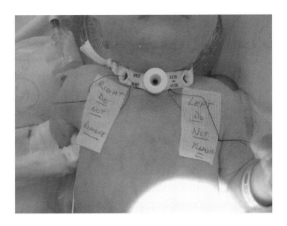

Figure 6.6 Tracheotomy tube in place with stay sutures labeled and taped to the chest. Take care to avoid crossing the stay sutures, as this mistake may complicate replacement of the tracheotomy tube in emergent situations.

The tracheotomy incision is not routinely packed or sutured to allow egress and to prevent subcutaneous emphysema. If it is anticipated that the tracheotomy will be permanent, then maturing sutures with absorbable material may be placed from the skin directly to the trachea.

Correct size and positioning of the tracheotomy tube can be confirmed with a post-operative chest radiograph and/or passage of a small pediatric flexible endoscope. The distal end of the tracheotomy tube should be 5–20 mm above the carina. Obtaining a chest film is advised to ensure that a pneumothorax did not occur intraoperatively. If the tracheotomy tube is too long, it may be cut to an appropriate size, while beveling sharp edges, until a special order tracheotomy tube can be obtained. Care must be taken not to shorten the tube too much as this may lead to posterior wall irritation or accidental decannulation. The Bivona adjustable length tube is an excellent temporary one to use when a special order tracheotomy tube is anticipated, such as an extra long one. Bivona tubes also have a connector extension option (Flex-tend, Portex[tm] products), which is very useful for children with short necks or redundant skin tissues.

Postoperative care

After tracheotomy, the patient should be closely monitored in the intensive care unit for 5–7 days. Humidification is provided through the ventilator circuit or via a tracheotomy collar and suctioning is performed as needed. Medical staff caring for the patient should be comfortable with the use of stay sutures in case of accidental decannulation. Feeding may be restarted within 1–2 days if other medical conditions allow.

Stomal maturation usually is complete after 5 days and the first tracheotomy tube change may be safely performed by the surgical team. Allowing time for the stoma to heal decreases the chances of placing the tracheotomy tube into false passages outside the tracheal lumen. During the first tube change, it is best if two individuals are present and the patient's neck extended with the use of a shoulder roll and adequate lighting. The original tube is removed, stoma wiped clean with sterile gauze, and the new tracheotomy tube is placed. Soft tracheotomy ties are placed snugly around the neck and stay sutures removed. Alternatively, tracheotomy tubes may be exchanged "over the wire" using a suction catheter or flexible endoscope. If the size of the tracheotomy tube is changed, an endoscope should be used to ensure appropriate positioning of the new tube.

Anesthetic management of tracheotomies

When approaching the preoperative assessment of a tracheotomy-dependent patient, some specific pieces of information must be identified beyond the routine pre-anesthetic interview. One must determine the underlying cause of respiratory failure responsible for the patient's tracheotomy dependence. This is crucial, as the anesthesiologist must know about the possibility of orotracheal intubation by conventional means in patients with tracheotomy secondary to a craniofacial syndrome. For those patients on home ventilators, it is important to know the extent of their ventilatory dependence, baseline ventilator settings, and any recent increases in their ventilator or oxygen requirements. Information should be obtained from the primary caregiver regarding the extent of oral secretions and suctioning needs to determine likelihood of a mucus plug. The tracheotomy stoma should be evaluated for issues such as erosion and granulation tissue, which may lead to bleeding or obstruction. Particular attention to the size and type of tracheotomy tube is important, assuring that replacements are available [7].

When approaching the intraoperative airway management of indwelling tracheotomies for surgical procedures, several options may be utilized depending on the particular nature and length of surgery, as well as the comfort level of the anesthesiologist.

(1) The tracheotomy may be left in place, recognizing the likely possibility of increased leak around the tube due to the decreased muscle tone under general anesthesia. If the procedure is not expected to be lengthy, ventilator settings may be increased to compensate for the leak, and a Tegaderm may be placed over the mouth and nose to decrease the extent of the leak. However, with this approach, end-tidal CO_2 monitoring may not be reliable, necessitating vigilance in following basic monitoring such as chest rise. Diligent organization of the anesthetic circuit is crucial, with the focus on preventing increased tension that may lead to an airway obstruction. If the decision has been made to maintain the tracheotomy in place, and the surgery proceeds for a time longer than expected, the anesthesiologist may want to consider obtaining a blood gas to determine CO_2 values more precisely.

(2) The uncuffed tracheotomy tube, commonly placed in smaller children, may be exchanged for a cuffed tube one-half size smaller. Positioning the patient properly, using neck extension, as well as generous lubrication of the tube, may allow easier exchange of the tracheotomy. Care must be taken to ensure that the shortened tube will not result in a cuff inflated at the tracheal stoma. If resistance is encountered upon attempts at inflation, a tracheotomy tube of the original size should be placed, minimally inflating the cuff enough to prevent a leak. The new tracheotomy tube may be secured with tape or the original cloth ties, avoiding excessive tightness upon fastening that might affect venous return.

(3) The tracheotomy tube may be exchanged for a well-lubricated, half-size smaller cuffed ETT. The ETT should be placed through the stoma until the cuff is no longer visible, then inflated to prevent a leak. The ETT should then be carefully taped or sutured to the chest wall.

(4) The tracheotomy tube may be replaced by an orally placed cuffed ETT, carefully assuring that the ETT cuff passes beyond the tracheal stoma. However, one must always be cognizant of the possibility of difficulty replacing the original tracheotomy at the end of the case due to stoma shrinkage.

It is important to remember that, in the event of an emergency, if you are unable to replace a tracheotomy tube, it is still possible to temporarily proceed with hand ventilation either through the stoma (infant mask over stoma while occluding mouth and nose) or through the mouth and nose (while occluding the stoma), while preparing alternative strategies to manage the airway. One should never force any tube through the tracheal stoma, due to concerns over forming a false passage near the trachea. Fiberoptic tracheoscopy with a flexible bronchoscope, placement of a guiding suction catheter, changing neck position, or even use of laryngoscope through the stoma may help facilitate placement of the tracheotomy tube or ETT without causing trauma, and possibly further complicating management of the airway. An important caveat; it would be prudent to consider early involvement of an otolaryngologist-head and neck surgeon, when difficulty is encountered in managing a patient with a tracheotomy, to prevent the development of an airway disaster [7].

When approaching the postoperative care of patients that are tracheotomy dependent, one must determine the most appropriate area for recovery (post-anesthesia care unit or intensive care unit), depending on the extent of surgery and patient's baseline ventilatory needs. In the post-anesthesia care unit, the patient may be placed on their own home ventilator with their baseline settings while recovering from anesthesia. Overnight stays are often appropriate, as the patient's respiratory drive may continue to be affected by residual medications and anesthetic [7].

Home care

Once the tracheotomy tube has been successfully changed, the patient may be transferred to the general medical floor and the parents or caregivers can be instructed in proper tracheotomy tube care and cardiopulmonary resuscitation. After the caregivers are trained and all the appropriate equipment is in place at the child's home, and the medical condition allows, the patient may be discharged home. The tracheotomy tube should be changed weekly and as needed if it becomes plugged with mucus. The caregivers should also have an emergency one-half size smaller tracheotomy tube available in case the stoma narrows making it difficult to replace the correct size. Local emergency response personnel should be alerted to the child's presence in the community, as well as the local telephone and electric companies, to give the child's home priority in cases when power is lost and repairs are needed.

Surveillance

There are disparate opinions regarding the appropriate timing and interval for post-tracheotomy surveillance or interval endoscopy. For children with rapidly evolving airway lesions, endoscopies are needed more frequently. Serial excisions or dilatations may be performed on a biweekly schedule for evolving lesions such as early subglottic stenosis. Young infants who are rapidly growing may also require frequent interval endoscopies. Interval endoscopies every 3–4 months to assess proper tube size is reasonable for such children. For children with stable airway lesions and long-term tracheotomies, biannual interval endoscopy is reasonable. For older teenagers with long-standing tracheotomies, a yearly endoscopy is warranted.

Immediate interval endoscopy is required for a child of any age if tracheotomy complications are suspected. Complications include significant bleeding, difficult tracheotomy tube change, false passage of the tube, aphonia, difficult suctioning, airway obstruction, pneumothorax, mucus plugging, atelectasis, and unexplained oxyhemoglobin desaturations, etc.

Early planned interventions are safer than rushed emergency procedures. Interval endoscopy is also warranted before possible decannulation to assess for unanticipated sources of airway obstruction, such as significant suprastomal collapse or obstructing granulation tissue.

Intraoperative complications

Hemorrhage

Appropriate history-taking should alert the physician to any pre-existing medical conditions that may lead to intraoperative hemorrhage such as hemophilia, von Willebrand disease, or renal failure. A medication history should be obtained to screen for any anticoagulant, aspirin, and/or non-steroidal anti-inflammatory use. Preoperative labs should check hemoglobin, platelets, and coagulation levels, and address any correctable abnormalities before surgery.

Careful dissection and ligature techniques are used for anterior jugular veins and the thyroid isthmus to avoid complications. Occasionally, local muscle flaps are used to cover larger vessels such as a high-riding innominate artery to allow for safe placement of the tracheotomy tube. It may also be necessary to remove the tracheotomy tube and replace the ETT, or bronchoscope to secure the airway to gain hemostasis before replacing the tracheotomy tube and leaving the operating suite.

Air dissection

Dissection of air into the deep paratracheal tissues may lead to pneumomediastinum, pneumothorax, or subcutaneous emphysema. This complication may be prevented by avoiding excessive dissection of the pretracheal fascia, securing the airway with an ETT before the procedure, and avoiding tight closure of the stomal skin to allow for air egress. Subcutaneous emphysema should resolve over time; however, occasionally, the skin incision needs to be widened or a chest tube is required.

Iatrogenic trauma

Identification of landmarks is essential to avoid damage to the cricoid cartilage that may lead to chondronecrosis and eventual subglottic stenosis. Optimal location for the tracheotomy incision is below the second tracheal ring. Limiting the dissection to midline will also help prevent injury to the recurrent laryngeal nerves, which lie within the tracheoesophageal groove. Care is also needed to prevent injury to the apical pleura, which in infants may extend into the inferior aspect of the neck leading to pneumothorax. During the tracheotomy incision, care should be taken to avoid inadvertent laceration of the posterior tracheal wall. Any laceration to the tracheoesophageal wall should be primarily repaired and may require a local muscle flap for optimal closure. Revision tracheotomy following previous tracheotomy or laryngotracheal reconstruction requires caution as the anatomy may be significantly distorted.

Tracheotomy tube problems

Appropriate positioning of the tracheotomy tube in the airway should be confirmed before leaving the operating room. If the distal port of the tracheotomy tube abuts the posterior tracheal wall, it may lead to difficulties in suctioning and obstruction. The length of the tube should be at least 5–20 mm proximal to the carina to avoid irritation and right main bronchus insertion. Passing a flexible endoscope through the tracheotomy tube, with the head in a neutral position, to ensure proper positioning may prevent these complications.

Postobstructive pulmonary edema

In the setting of chronic or subacute airway obstruction, the sudden release of these forces followed by laryngospasm may result in high intrathoracic negative pressures leading to flash pulmonary edema. The increased interstitial pulmonary fluid may be relieved with diuretics and positive pressure ventilation.

Early postoperative complications

Hemorrhage

Early postoperative bleeding may be due to underlying coagulopathy or to vasoconstrictive effects of local anesthetics wearing off. Minimal oozing may be controlled with light packing of the incision with care taken to avoid displacement of the tracheotomy tube and air trapping. If the bleeding is more severe or does not respond to conservative measures then returning to the operating room for exploration is warranted.

Wound infection

Colonization typically occurs within 24 h of a tracheotomy; however, occasionally, local cellulitis, tracheitis, or frank pneumonia may ensue. Although sterile technique is employed while performing the tracheotomy, infections often occur due to the clean-contaminated nature of airway surgery. Culture- and sensitivity-directed antibiotic administration is advised as infecting agents are often resistant to first-line antimicrobials. In addition, the discovery of biofilms in the tube lumen of has further complicated the treatment of tracheotomy site infections [8].

Dysphagia

The tethering effect of the tracheotomy tube to the skin may prevent adequate laryngeal elevation leading to dysphagia. In addition, the laryngeal closure reflex is often impaired due to the lack of airflow stimulation past the true vocal folds. Aspiration may result from inadequate laryngeal closure during the pharyngeal swallowing phase. Although cuffed tracheotomy tubes and suctioning may decrease the amount of aspiration, increased cuff pressure may impair esophageal food passage, further exacerbating aspiration. Continuous positive airway pressure has been used to prevent chronic salivary aspiration in certain individuals [9]; however, intractable aspiration is treated with laryngotracheal separation procedures.

Obstruction of the tracheotomy tube

Tracheotomy tubes may obstruct if they are too short and abut the posterior tracheal wall. If they are too long, they may touch the anterior tracheal wall. Ensuring proper positioning of the tube within the tracheal lumen with flexible endoscopy can prevent this complication. Thick tenacious mucus or blood may also plug tracheotomy tubes. Adequate humidification and the use of heat moisture exchangers and appropriate suctioning reduce the incidence of mucus plugging. The inner cannulas of tracheotomy tubes should be changed and cleaned frequently. Those tubes without inner cannulas should be changed on a weekly basis to avoid obstruction.

Accidental decannulation

During the first 5–7 days after surgery, accidental decannulation may be life threatening, as the tracheal stoma is not yet mature. Close observation in the intensive care unit in the postoperative period is recommended to prevent the patient from manipulating the tracheotomy tube and potentially causing decannulation. Occasionally, sedation is necessary for patients who are extremely active. Tracheotomy ties should be fixed circumferentially around the neck allowing only one finger's breadth between the skin and the tie. Some also advocate suturing the tracheotomy flange directly to the skin until the first tube change, although this may make removal and replacement of a tube in the paratracheal position more difficult. In accidental decannulation, proper use of the traction sutures is imperative to replace the tracheotomy tube safely. Gentle anterior and lateral retraction, without crossing the sutures, is necessary to open the tracheotomy site successfully. Alternative techniques in replacing tracheotomy tubes include passing the tube over a suction catheter or flexible bronchoscope. One should also always have a tube available one-half size smaller for cases of stomal stenosis. If the tracheotmy tube cannot be quickly replaced, alternatives must be immediately found to supply oxygen such as mask ventilation for intubation via the upper airway.

Late postoperative complications

Granuloma formation

Suprastomal granulomas typically form at the superior aspect of the internal tracheal stoma. These lesions may cause difficulties in tracheotomy tube changes, bleed, or dislodge causing dangerous distal obstructions. Small, soft granulomas may be removed transstomally with hooks and hemostats, coblation [10], or microdebridement. Alternatively, they may be removed with KTP (potassium titanyl phosphate) or YAG lasers passed through a bronchoscope. When granulomas are very large, they may require open excision. Granulomas may obstruct a significant portion of the airway and should be addressed before attempting to decannulate. Some physicians advocate removal of only large granulomas or granulomas present before decannulation, as granuloma removal has been shown to increase the risk of recurrence [11].

Suprastomal collapse

Collapse of the tracheal rings above the level of the tracheotomy site is a common complication after tracheotomy. Vertical tracheal incisions during the initial tracheotomy help to reduce the incidence of this problem. The posterior and superior aspects of the tracheotomy tube press against the anterior tracheal surface, weakening and causing retrodisplacement of the cartilaginous tracheal rings, which may result in stenosis. This obstruction may be severe enough to prevent successful decannulation. In these cases the collapsed segment may require surgical excision (endoscopic or open) or reconstruction with cartilage grafting.

Tracheoesophageal fistula

Delayed tracheoesphageal fistula may result from ischemic necrosis of the posterior trachea often due to an overinflated tracheotomy tube cuff and a large bore nasogastric tube. Small fistulas may be treated with removal of the tubes and wound drainage. Larger fistulas may require direct closure with muscle flaps.

Tracheal and subglottic stenosis

Airway stenosis secondary to tracheotomy tube placement may occur at various levels. The subglottis, suprastomal, stomal, cuff region, and distal port may develop stenosis, which may be exacerbated by infectious processes and gastroesophageal reflux. High tracheotomy incisions predispose to subglottic stenosis by injury to the cricoid cartilage. Posterior displacement of the superior tracheal rings and granuloma formation cause suprastomal collapse. Excessive pressure within the tracheotomy tube cuff will lead to ischemic injury to the surrounding mucosa and potentially cause chondritis leading to tracheal stenosis. Local trauma from the tracheotomy tube tip may also damage the tracheal lumen resulting in scar tissue formation.

When diagnosed early, stenosis of the trachea responds well to corticosteroids, antibiotics, and acid suppression. Small mature stenosis may require serial dilations or laser excisions while lesions that are more extensive require open surgical reconstruction with rib grafts or reanastomosis.

Tracheoinnominate artery fistula

Erosion of the innominate artery by the tracheotomy tube is often heralded by a "sentinel bleed" in which a patient coughs up a small amount of bright red blood before a massive arterial hemorrhage. This complication may result from: (1) placing the tracheotomy incision too low in the neck, which allows the distal port of the tube to contact the anterior tracheal wall at the level of the innominate artery; (2) an aberrant course of the artery, which is too high; (3) a poor fitting tube, which is too long and irritates the anterior tracheal wall; (4) overinflated tracheotomy cuff pressure, which erodes through the trachea; (5) and infection, which erodes through the trachea into the innominate artery.

When tracheoinnominate fistulas occur, time is not a luxury and skilled medical attention is required for optimal patient outcomes. The patient should be transported to the operating suite for bronchoscopy. If a fistula is identified a cuffed ETT is passed such that the cuff is adjacent to the bleeding. The ETT cuff is maximally inflated and suprasternal pressure is applied to tamponade the bleeding. Blood transfusions are administered as needed and a sternotomy is performed to access the innominate artery for control. Performing these maneuvers increases the patient's survival from 7% to 50% [12].

Persistent tracheocutaneous fistula

Failure of spontaneous tracheocutaneous fistula closure following decannulation occurs when mature epithelium lines the stomal tract. This complication is more common in mature tracheotomy sites and after a "starplasty" tracheotomy technique [13]. Fistulae are closed by excising the epithelial tract and allowing the wound to heal via secondary intention.

A Penrose drain is placed allowing any air to escape preventing subcutaneous emphysema. Close observation for subcutaneous emphysema is required after tracheocutaneous fistula closure.

Outcomes

Decannulation

Feasibility of decannulation and a timeframe within which to proceed with decannulation may depend on original indications for placement of the tracheotomy. Reported rates of decannulation vary, ranging from 29% to 98% [2], and are greatly impacted by the patient population of each particular case series. Both an increased time to decannulation and reduced overall success in decannulation may be expected in those patients with neurological impairment or prolonged intubation. However, decannulation may be more successful and occur within a significantly shorter timeframe in those patients receiving tracheotomies due to craniofacial anomalies [14]. In general, however, the rate of successful decannulation has decreased, and the retention time of the tracheal stoma has more than doubled to greater than 2 years [2]. This might be attributed to changing indications for pediatric tracheotomy; specifically, the performance of fewer short-term tracheotomies for acute infections, as well as advances in neonatal medicine allowing for long-term tracheotomies in severely compromised children. Children who are decannulated within 2 years of placement of the tracheotomy are less likely to develop a tracheocutaneous fistula [14].

Mortality

The mortality rate for pediatric patients with a tracheotomy has been reported as two to three times higher than in the adult population, yet may vary by as much as 40% depending on the case series [15]. An overwhelming majority of deaths in these patients are ascribed to the child's primary illness [14]. Many studies also indicate an increased mortality rate among children receiving tracheotomies below 1 year of age, likely related to distinct pathologies within the particular patient population [15]. Tracheotomy-related mortality ranges from 0% to 6% [14,15] and may be altered by a number of factors, including the number of

Table 6.2 The standard supplies for a patient discharged to home with tracheotomy tube (Boig CW. *Children's Hospital of Pittsburgh Tracheostomy Care Procedures Manual.* Personal Communication, 2009)

Standard tracheotomy supplies for home care	
Humidifier	Resuscitation bag – reusable
Suction – portable	Resuscitation bag – disposable
Suction – stationary	Tubing circuits
Suction catheters	Tracheotomy tubes
Pulse – oximeter	Tracheotomy tube ties
Pulse – ox probes	Normal saline solution

operations performed by the surgeon, number of tracheotomized children treated at the hospital, as well as specialization of the hospital. Pediatric hospitals with interdisciplinary care and multiple tracheotomies performed within a single department contribute greatly to reduced mortality [16].

Speech and language development

Patients with tracheotomies have been shown to exhibit difficulties with speech and language development, even after decannulation. In children with a primary neurologic disorder, the difficulties they experience are largely related to the primary disease process. However, even in patients without a neurologic disorder, tracheotomy itself contributes to speech impairment by inhibiting vocalization and language development. The aphonia imposed by the tracheotomy and absence of auditory and oral–motor biofeedback may be compounded by reduced language stimulation from the primary caregivers [17]. Even those patients with optimal outcomes may still have developmental problems, such as slower growth rate and behavioral issues, requiring intervention by special education and/or rehabilitation programs [18]. Age at tracheotomy and decannulation may play a significant role in long-term language ability. Patients receiving tracheotomy at an older age, after which the fundamentals of language have already been implanted, as well as those patients with a shorter length of cannulation, may have less adverse consequences [19]. Similarly, children decannulated during the prelinguistic stage of childhood maintain speech and language skills commensurate with intellectual ability, whereas decannulation during the linguistic stage may lead to phonologic impairment. However, even those patients exhibiting language skills on par with their intellectual abilities may still have expressive language disability secondary to their tracheotomy [17]. Recommendations for decannulation before 15 months may lead to the best possible outcome for speech and language development [19]. Tracheotomy speaking valves may present another option for voice production while the tracheotomy is still in place.

Conclusions

The case of semi-emergent tracheotomy presented at the beginning of the chapter illustrates several important points regarding the importance of planning and communication between the Intensive Care Unit, Anesthesia, and Otolaryngology Departments. The Intensive Care Department provided the necessary initial medical therapy and supportive care. When the stridor and airway obstruction progressed, they wisely alerted the Anesthesia and Otolaryngology Departments in time to allow transfer of the patient to the operating room before the child progressed to total airway obstruction or respiratory arrest from fatigue. The anesthesiolgist maintained ventilation and provided the anesthestic to allow a safe and thorough evaluation of the airway by the Otolaryngologist with the rigid bronchoscope. When the Otolaryngologist diagnosed a severe subglottic stenosis and the child progressed to oxyhemoglobin desaturation, the bronchoscope was safely passed to secure the airway, save the child's life and allow an orderly, uncomplicated tracheotomy over the bronchoscope. This thoughtful team approach and communication between services is essential for management of these critical life-threatening airway issues.

Tracheostomy is a lifesaving procedure that demands an intimate understanding of the indications, anatomy and technique, peri- and post- operative care, and potential complications. This is especially true in the pediatric population. Although the indications have changed since Habicot performed the first life-saving pediatric tracheotomy, many things have remained the same. Proper training, a careful and thoughtful team approach, and excellent post-tracheotomy care is required for optimal patient outcomes.

References

1. Pereira KD, MacGregor AR, McDuffie CM, Mitchell RB. Tracheostomy in preterm infants. *Arch Otolaryngol Head Neck Surg* 2003; **129**: 1268–71.

2. Zenk J, Fyrmpas G, Zimmermann T, Koch M, Constantinidis J, Iro H. Tracheostomy in young patients: indications and long-term outcome. *Eur Arch Otorhinolaryngol* 2009; **266**: 705–11.

3. Graf JM, Montagnino BA, Hueckel R, McPherson ML. Pediatric tracheostomies: a recent experience from one academic center. *Pediatr Crit Care Med* 2008; **9**: 96–100.

4. Hopkins C, Whetstone S, Foster T, Blaney S, Morrison G. The impact of paediatric tracheostomy on both patient and parent. *Int J Pediatr Otorhinolaryngol* 2009; **73**: 15–20.

5. Yellon RF. Technique and complications of tracheostomy in the pediatric age group. In: Myers EN, Johnson JT, eds. *Tracheotomy. Airway Management, Communication, and Swallowing*, 2nd edition. San Diego: Plural Publishing, 2008; 69–82.

6. Isaacson G. In: Bluestone CD, Casselbrant ML, Stool SE, *et al.*, eds. *Pediatric Otolaryngology* 4th edn. Philadelphia: Saunders. 2003; chp 74: 1361–70.

7. Ross P. Anesthesia for the pediatric patient with a tracheostomy. *Semin Anesth Periop Med Pain* 2007; **26**: 153–7.

8. Perkins J, Mouzakes J, Pereira R, Manning S. Bacterial biofilm presence in pediatric tracheostomy tubes. *Arch Otolaryngol Head Neck Surg* 2004; **130**(3): 339–43.

9. Finder JD, Yellon RF, Charron M. Successful management of tracheostomized patients with chronic salivary aspiration by use of constant positive airway pressure. *Pediatrics* 2001; **107**(6): 1343–5.

10. Kitsko DJ, Chi DH. Coblation removal of large suprastomal granulomas. *Laryngoscope* 2009; **119**(2): 387–9.

11. Rosenfeld RM, Stool SE. Should granulomas be excised in children with long term tracheostomy? *Arch Otolaryngol Head Neck Sur* 1992; **118**(12): 1323–7.

12. Jones JW, Reynolds M, Hewitt RL, Drapanas T. Tracheoinnominant artery erosion: successful surgical management of a devastating complication. *Ann Surg* 1976; **184**(2): 194–204.

13. Sautter NB, Krakovitz PR, Solares CA, Koltai PJ. Closure of persistent tracheocutaneous fistula following "starplasty" tracheostomy in children. *Int J Pediatr Otorhinolaryngol* 2006; **70**: 99–105.

14. Carron JD, Derkay CS, Strope GL, Nosonchuk JE, Darrow DH. Pediatric tracheostomies: changing indications and outcomes. *Laryngoscope* 2000; **110**(7): 1099–104.

15. Kremer B, Botos-Kremer AI, Eckel HE, Schlondorff G. Indications, complications, and surgical techniques for pediatric tracheostomies – an update. *J Pediatr Surg* 2002; **37**: 1556–62.

16. Lewis CW, Carron JD, Perkins JA, Sie KC, Feudtner C. Tracheotomy in pediatric patients: a national perspective. *Arch Otolaryngol Head Neck Surg* 2003; **129**: 523–9.

17. Hill BP, Singer LT. Speech and language development after infant tracheostomy. *J Speech Hearing Disord* 1990; **55**: 15–20.

18. Singer LT, Kercsmar C, Legris G, Orlowski JP, Hill BP, Doershuk C. Developmental sequelae of long-term infant tracheostomy. *Dev Med Child Neurol* 1989; **31**: 224–30.

19. Jiang D, Morrison GAJ. The influence of long-term tracheostomy on speech and language development in children. *Int J Pediatr Otorhinolaryngol* 2003; **67S1**: S217–20.

Laryngotracheal reconstruction: surgical management of pediatric airway stenosis

Diego Preciado, Sophie R. Pestieau, and Ira Todd Cohen

Case presentation

Case 1

A 4-month-old premature (26 weeks' gestation) male infant, with laryngotracheal stenosis has had several failed attempts at extubation. Previous medical history is remarkable for a complicated neonatal course, including sepsis, surgical closure of a patent ductus arteriosus, grade IV intraventricular hemorrhage, and retinopathy of prematurity.

Case 2

A 2-year-old child with a tracheotomy, secondary to subglottic stenosis (SGS), stridor, and failure to thrive, is scheduled for a laryngotracheal reconstruction. Medical history is remarkable for reactive airway disease, gastroesophageal reflux, and multiple admissions (one intensive care unit) for respiratory distress. Home medications include albuterol, budesonide, montelukast, and lansoprazole.

Introduction

The management of laryngotracheal stenosis in children poses multiple challenges for clinicians. The severity of subglottic stenosis (SGS) can vary greatly. The grading scale most universally employed was proposed by Myer *et al.* in 1994 using percentage of narrowing: grade 1, 0–50%; grade 2, 50–75%; grade 3, 75–99%; and grade 4, no identifiable lumen [1]. Although avoiding tracheotomy or achieving decannulation can be expected at a rate of approximately 90% [2–5], success rates in children with severe stenosis are lower [3,6,7]. A single, uniform, open procedure to reconstruct the narrowed pediatric airway does not exist but, in general, open airway reconstruction is indicated when the stenosis is mature, circumferential, long, greater than 50%, or failing to resolve with simple endoscopic techniques such as balloon dilation. The open airway laryngotracheal reconstruction (LTR) procedures available to the airway surgeon include anterior cricoid split (ACS), laryngotracheoplasty

Tracheotomy Management: A Multidisciplinary Approach, ed. Peggy A. Seidman, David Goldenberg and Elizabeth H. Sinz. Published by Cambridge University Press. © Cambridge University Press 2011.

(LTP) with cartilage grafting, and partial cricotracheal resection (pCTR). A brief description of these, including their indications will be covered in this chapter.

Any of the above procedures can be done in a "single-stage" or "double-stage" approach. "Single-stage" procedures refer to those where there is no tracheotomy postoperatively. These are typically performed in patients with healthy lungs and isolated, simple stenotic lesions. For patients with multilevel or more severe pathologies, including previously failed reconstructive attempts, or in those where "single-stage" procedures are contraindicated due to poor pulmonary reserve, a tracheotomy tube is left in place postoperatively. Patients require a second procedure (decannulation) hence the role as a "double-stage" approach.

The use of postoperative tracheal stenting plays an important designation in the surgical management of these patients and is used regardless of the LTR procedure performed (ACS versus LTR versus pCTR). Stenting is imperative to maintain cartilage grafts in position, lend support to the reconstructed or anastomosed area, and to provide a rigid luminal framework around which healing and scar contracture can occur. For those patients where "single-stage" surgery is performed short-term stenting with nasotracheal intubation in the pediatric intensive care unit (PICU) for 5–10 days is usually sufficient. For those patients where "double-stage" procedures are performed, longer-term postoperative stenting is accomplished with indwelling suprastomal laryngotracheal stents.

Preoperative considerations

Patients undergoing LTR, such as those presented above, frequently have complex medical histories and concurrent disorders. The preoperative evaluation should include a detailed history and physical assessment. Most infants with acquired SGS will have had a history of neonatal intubation [8,9]. Patients presently and formerly in the neonatal intensive care unit need careful cardiopulmonary assessment and evaluation for any congenital abnormalities. Difficulties with airway management and intravenous access should be anticipated. Baseline laboratory values such as hematocrit, hemoglobin, electrolytes, should be noted, and oxygen saturation should be obtained.

As in Case 2, sequelae of long-standing airway compromise may lead to or be related to other organ system disorders. The severity of reactive airway disease needs to be evaluated and treatment with bronchodilators and glucocorticoids should be optimized before surgery. Possible concomitant gastroesophageal reflux (GERD) should be investigated and treated, as many have reported a correlation between presence of GERD and severe SGS [10,11], and GERD may affect surgical healing after LTR [12,13]. Patients with dysphagia, or severe laryngeal and hypopharyngeal inflammation should be evaluated for eosinophilic esophagitis, as this emerging disorder has also recently been shown to be associated with SGS and can negatively influence on healing and outcomes after LTR [14,15]. As above, baseline laboratory values should be obtained. Preoperative radiographic imaging plays little to no role in anesthetic or surgical planning except to help characterize and determine chronic lung parenchyma changes and the length of a stenotic airway segment.

The ideal timing of LTR surgery remains somewhat ill-defined. Some have demonstrated that children younger than 24 months have higher rates of reconstruction failure despite lesser degrees of stenotic pathology when compared with older children [16]. More recent larger series have shown that although younger children have a higher rate of reintubation after single-stage procedures, eventually they can be extubated, and that age alone is not a predictor for reconstructive failure (defined as failure to decannulate or avoid tracheotomy) [1,2,6].

In children with existing tracheotomies, LTR timing decisions must consider that severe SGS managed with tracheotomy, where formal LTR is deferred, is potentially life threatening as yearly tracheotomy-specific mortality in children due to tracheotomy tube obstruction is 1–3.4% [17–19]. Associated tracheotomy tube morbidity also includes the need for comprehensive nursing care and monitoring, delayed speech and language development, feeding difficulties, and infection. Therefore, many authors now propose reconstruction as early as possible to avoid prolonged tracheotomy [1,2,6,20].

Undoubtedly, the gold standard in the preoperative airway evaluation and SGS characterization is a rigid direct laryngoscopy and bronchoscopy (DLB) procedure under general anesthesia. Most commonly, anesthetic management for this evaluation is accomplished in children using spontaneous ventilation with a mixture of sevoflurane and oxygen for induction and infusion of propofol or other intravenous agents and insufflation of oxygen for maintenance of anesthesia. This approach allows dynamic assessment of the laryngotracheobronchial tree while manipulating the airway without needing intubation or ventilation through a rigid bronchoscope. The surgeon is simply able to use narrow rigid fiberoptic "naked" telescopes for diagnostic purposes, minimizing airway trauma associated with the larger diameter ventilating bronchoscope. The ventilating bronchoscope is then reserved for cases where therapeutic or interventional maneuvers have to be performed in the trachea and mainstem bronchi. After DLB is performed, to objectively determine severity of the stenosis the lumen of the stenotic airway is typically sized using an endotracheal tube (ETT) [7].

Flexible laryngobronchoscopy is complementary to rigid DLB and helps to assess the degree of possible obstruction at the tongue base in patients with severe micrognathia, and to reach distal aspects of the bronchial tree. Flexible laryngobronchoscopy is also best accomplished without intubation, under spontaneous ventilation with oxygen insufflation through the side port of the flexible scope. This approach allows the endoscopist not to be limited on having to perform flexible endoscopy without an ETT, the lumen of which in infants is often too small to allow for passage of a flexible scope with suction capability.

For patients with laryngotracheal stenosis without an existing tracheotomy tube, further and definitive reconstructive management is based upon the clinical picture and severity of the stenotic segment. The presence of chronic pulmonary disease, often represented by baseline oxygen requirement in bronchopulmonary dysplasia and poor pulmonary functional reserve, prohibits single-stage LTR, necessitating placement of a tracheotomy before or during the LTR.

Intraoperative management

Anesthetic management

Induction and maintenance of anesthesia for LTR requires careful preparation for and attention to airway management and overall homeostasis. The room should be warmed for these infants and toddlers who can quickly cool; standard monitors, including precordial stethoscope, pulse oximetry, electrocardiogram, non-invasive blood pressure, end-tidal CO_2, and temperature probe, are the minimum requirement for otherwise healthy patients. Invasive blood pressure monitor and easy access to arterial blood gas sampling are advisable for patients with significant pulmonary or cardiac disease. A full assortment of ETT and laryngoscope blade sizes and types, as well as suction catheters, stylets, and handles, should be readily available.

By preserving spontaneous respiration during induction, DLB is often the only way of maintaining adequate ventilation. Significantly stenosed airways may offer marked resistance to positive pressure ventilation. Achieving an anesthesia depth for these highly stimulating procedures without suppressing respiratory drive can be difficult, especially in sick or small infants. High doses of general anesthetics can be avoided by using topical anesthesia (i.e., 4 mg/kg of 2–4% lidocaine) sprayed on the larynx and vocal cords. The lower concentration of lidocaine is sometimes preferred in smaller infants because it is easier to control the dose. Although dexamethasone is often given for routine DLB its administration should be delayed to a later time in the postoperative period before extubation, to avoid interfering with wound healing. After DLB and airway sizing, endotracheal intubation will be performed and the ETT secured. The head and airway must remain accessible for repeat laryngotracheal assessments by the otolaryngologist-head and neck surgeon and eventual placement of the postoperative artificial airway.

To avoid contamination of the surgical theater with anesthetic gases, total intravenous anesthesia can be used for anesthetic maintenance. For single-stage procedures, with planned prolonged postoperative intubation and sedation, a technique is suggested that will minimize the onset of tolerance to commonly used sedatives and analgesics. With the combination of opioids, low-dose ketamine, and α_2 agonists, pain can be alleviated while reducing the onset of opioid-induced tolerance and hyperalgesia. Other agents to consider for supplemental anesthesia and perioperative sedation are propofol and benzodiazepines. Once the airway is repaired and there is minimal to no leak of anesthetic gases, volatile agents such as sevoflurane can safely be administered. This multimodal pharmacologic approach provides an effective and safe intraoperative anesthetic management in infants and children who are at high risk for tolerance to opioids and sedatives.

Patients undergoing LTR may require analgesia for a minimum 7–10 days, leading to large doses of opioids to treat pain. Tolerance to opioids and opioid-induced hyperalgesia are possible explanations for escalating opioid requirements and inadequacy of pain control. Activation of N-methyl-D-aspartate receptors by μ-receptor agonists has been assumed as one of the underlying mechanisms [21–23]. Low-dose ketamine has been shown to be beneficial in the management of acute postoperative pain after a variety of surgical procedures [23–25]. A previous literature review has shown that to be effective in decreasing opioid consumption, ketamine needs to be given before the initial surgical stimulus, followed by an intraoperative and postoperative infusion [24]. Clinical side effects of ketamine at these low doses are unreported. Experimental data demonstrate increased apoptosis in the developing brain [26,27] and should be avoided in infants less than 6 months of age, as in Case 1.

Dexmedetomidine is a selective α_2-adrenoreceptor agonist that provides sedation, amnesia, and analgesia without respiratory depression [28,29]. Dexmedetomidine produces dose-dependent sympatholytic effects, including decreases in blood pressure and heart rate because of its α_2 adrenoreceptor agonist effects on the sympathetic ganglia [30,31]. However, its high α_2 receptor selectivity provides more hemodynamic stability than seen with clonidine, making it an attractive agent in these infants and children who may have other comorbidities. Although there are still many ongoing trials determining the safety of dexmedetomidine in children, it has been described as a useful, safe adjunct in many clinical applications, including sedation and rapid weaning in the intensive care unit [32,33]. Dexmedetomidine has also been shown to decrease postoperative opioid usage by more than 50%. Therefore, it may be a useful adjunct in the perioperative management of infants and children undergoing LTR.

For the double-stage procedure where a tracheotomy is placed before or during LTR, the tracheotomy tube will remain postoperatively, allowing for prompt awakening at the end of surgery or shortly thereafter. These infants and children may have a similar anesthetic as the single-stage procedure, but the postoperative course will be a lot more elementary in regards to sedation and analgesia.

Surgical management

Endoscopic treatment

In general, endoscopic treatment is limited to acquired (and not congenital) airway stenoses. Classically, endoscopic treatment has taken the form of laser ablation of narrowing lesions, but is only useful for non-mature, non-circumferential, short soft lesions that comprise mild grade 1 or 2 stenoses [34,35]. Recent small case series have also described balloon dilating catheters as potential tools that may successfully treat some patients with SGS, even if severe. [36,37] Larger studies are necessary to validate this approach. In any circumstance, dilation may certainly help temporize obstructive symptoms. Multiple, serial repeated dilations might eventually weaken the airway lateral walls, making the pathology worse.

Anterior cricoid split

The ACS procedure was introduced by Cotton and Seid in 1980 as an alternative approach to tracheotomy in premature neonates who have healthy lungs but failed extubation secondary to laryngeal obstruction arising from edema and early stenosis [38]. To qualify for this procedure, the only reason for extubation failure must be laryngeal obstruction. The neonate should have grown to 1.5 kg, required no assisted ventilatory support for 10 days, have no supplemental oxygen need greater than an FiO_2 of 35%, and have no evidence of congestive heart failure. The procedure consists of making an anterior vertical split through the first tracheal ring, cricoid cartilage, and lower thyroid cartilage followed by nasotracheal intubation for 10–14 days in NICU. If criteria are followed, case series have demonstrated ACS to be successful in avoiding tracheotomy in the majority of neonates [20]. During ACS, placement of a small piece of thyroid ala cartilage into the vertical split has also been described [39] and some claim it can improve the success of the surgery [40] (Figure 7.1).

Laryngotracheoplasty with cartilage grafting

LTP with interposition of cartilage graft was introduced by Fearon and Cotton in 1972 [41] as a means to expand an otherwise narrowed subglottic airway segment. The principle of the procedure is to distract the cricoid cartilage either anteriorly and/or posteriorly by suturing cartilaginous grafts in place over a luminal, appropriately sized stent.

In single-stage LTP procedures, the stent used is an ETT, which is left in place while the child is nasotracheally intubated and sedated in PICU for 5–14 days. Large outcome studies demonstrate success (defined by avoidance of tracheotomy need) of single-stage LTP surgery in over 80% of children [2]. The only factor associated with surgical failure was the presence of tracheomalacia. Management of the child in the postoperative period while intubated in PICU is often difficult and continually evolving. Reports suggest that older children (>3 years old) tolerate the intubation period better and often require minimal sedation or ventilatory assistance [42].

In double-stage procedures, a tracheotomy tube is either placed or left in place after surgery. As a stent, a sutured indwelling suprastomal stent is left in place postoperatively while grafts heal. Usually the stents are left in place for 2–6 weeks. Double-stage approaches are necessary when the child needs prolonged stenting, more complex airway lesions,

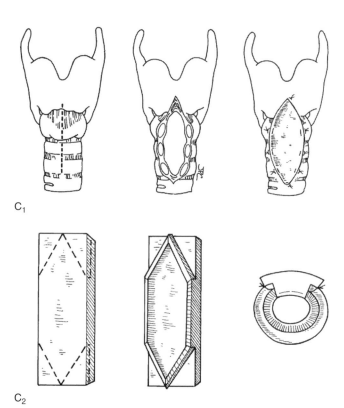

Figure 7.1 Anterior cricoid split.

C_1

C_2

concomitant airway pathology (such as tracheomalacia or tongue base obstruction), or in revision surgical cases. In cases when the reconstructed tracheal walls are flaccid, or there is poor graft stability, or if the anatomy is highly distorted due to previous multiple failed reconstruction attempts, stenting for longer than 6 weeks is warranted. Traditionally in adults, the most commonly used long-term laryngotracheal stent has been the Montgomery T-tube. Recently, it has also been shown to be an effective, reliable stent in children [43] allowing long-term stenting (>2 months). T-tubes provide stable, long-term laryngeal stenting with the possibility of vocalization. However, due to possible increased problems with obstruction and aspiration, they are restricted to children older than 4 years of age.

Cricotracheal resection

Resection of a narrowed laryngotracheal airway segment was first introduced in adults by Conley in 1953 [44] and later popularized in children by Monnier in the 1990s [45]. Multiple reports have since demonstrated that this procedure is more likely to achieve decannulation or avoid a tracheotomy tube in children with severe grade 3 or grade 4 stenosis [1,46–48], where success rates of greater than 90% have been reported. The concept of this procedure is to resect the narrowed subglottic airway, including the anterolateral cricoid cartilage ring, sparing the posterior cricoid cartilaginous plate, and maintaining functional cricoarytenoid joints. As with LTP procedures, CTR can be done in a single- or double-stage fashion. Additional postoperative considerations include using chin-to-chest sutures for 7–10 days to prevent neck extension and anastomotic dehiscence (Figure 7.2).

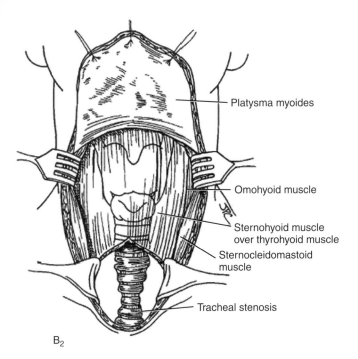

Platysma myoides

Omohyoid muscle

Sternohyoid muscle
over thyrohyoid muscle

Sternocleidomastoid
muscle

Tracheal stenosis

B₂

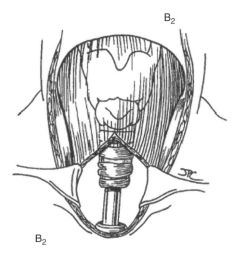

B₂

B₂

Displace endotracheal
tube laterally to effect
post sutures

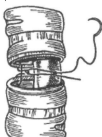
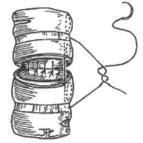
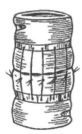

C

Figure 7.2 Segmental tracheal resection.

Postoperative considerations

Postoperative considerations for patients undergoing laryngotracheal reconstructive procedures depend on the nature of the surgery. For those patients undergoing single-stage procedures, endotracheal intubation is essential to allow healing and prevent airway obstruction associated with postoperative edema [49]. These infants and children will remain electively intubated in PICU for several days after surgery, thus requiring deep levels of sedation and analgesia. During this period, the use of sedation protocols is likely to be helpful in minimizing complications. Children that require high doses of sedation, paralytic agents, and controlled, assisted ventilation are at higher risk of pneumonia, withdrawal, and need for reintubation. These morbidities are especially salient in young neonates and children less than 3 years of age. Older children are less likely to require high levels of ventilatory and anesthetic support. The use of physical and pharmacologic restraints after single-stage LTR varies with age and mental development. Jacobs and colleagues showed that older developmentally appropriate children who were not sedated or restrained and who were allowed liberal physical activity had shorter lengths of stay in PICU and hospital, and a decreased incidence of postoperative adverse events [42]. In children 3 years old and older, it is possible to consider a postoperative management strategy that avoids sedatives, muscle relaxants, and physical restraints, and allows liberal bedside physical activity.

In younger children and infants, sedation and analgesia are necessary to prevent excessive head and neck movement with potential tension on the tracheal anastomosis. Immobility is also crucial to minimize movement of the indwelling ETT that may result in the disruption of suture lines or cause injury to the tracheal mucosa. Other goals of providing adequate sedation and analgesia in these children include alleviating pain, managing opioid-induced tolerance, and preventing opioid-induced hyperalgesia. Specific agents used to manage sedation and analgesia, as well as guidance as to their optimal use in the context of LTR, were discussed earlier in this chapter. Drug doses may be determined most appropriately using validated scoring tools for sedation and analgesia; these scales continue to evolve and are used with increasing regularity in PICU. Monitoring sedation along with the judicial use of sedation, analgesics, N-methyl-D-aspartate antagonists, α_2-adrenoreceptor agonists, and other pharmacological adjuncts are essential in providing a multimodal regimen.

Neuromuscular blockade to ensure patient safety remains controversial. Continuous neuromuscular blockade has been advocated in infants and young children to avoid ETT trauma to the fresh graft and potentially life-threatening accidental decannulation. Pulmonary atelectasis is the most common morbidity associated with prolonged neuromuscular blockade. Neuromuscular weakness also may follow prolonged paralysis and prolong hospitalization. The question remains whether postoperative management of such patients can be done safely and effectively without using paralyzing agents in the postoperative period. Bauman and colleagues compared the postoperative course of 17 patients who underwent a single-stage LTR [50, 51]. Half of the patients received continuous neuromuscular blockade while the other half was managed with daily 4–8-hour "interruptions" of paralysis. Overall these patients had less atelectasis and were extubated sooner than patients receiving continuous neuromuscular blockade. Intermittent paralysis or no paralysis also allows a more accurate pain assessment. In the absence of neuromuscular blockade, diligent nursing care with adequate sedation and analgesia is necessary to avoid the risk of accidental extubation.

Complex sedation and pain management post-LTR may not be needed in developmentally appropriate children over 2 years of age. Jacobs and colleagues reported that older children who were not sedated or restrained, and allowed physical activity had less postoperative adverse events and a shorter length of stay [42].

For double-stage patients, meticulous care of the tracheotomy tube is mandatory. This is particularly important if a suprastomal stent is above the tracheotomy tube making the child completely tube dependent for an airway. In this setting, accidental decannulation or tracheotomy mucus plugging are potentially lethal events. Given that children with suprastomal stents, and certainly those with Montgomery T-tubes, are likely to aspirate to a varying degree, a risk of pneumonia also exists. Cooperation with a speech and language pathologist to gauge the child's ability to swallow or aspiration risk is critical in postoperative double-stage patients with indwelling stents.

Conclusions

The two cases described at the beginning of the chapter were handled using different techniques. The four-month-old baby was brought to operating room from the NICU intubated with an uncuffed 2.5 mm endotracheal tube (ETT), FiO2 50% and SpO2 96%. A cricoid split was performed, complicated by minor bleeding from site, which was cauterized and controlled with minimal difficulty. He returned to the neonatal intensive care unit with an ETT in place. After five days he was extubated and given nasal CPAP. He continued to do well and was discharged three weeks later.

The two-year-old child was admitted preoperatively to optimize pulmonary function prior to surgery. In the operating room, anesthesia was induced using a potent inhalational agent via the existing tracheotomy and intravenous access was obtained. Using a flexible fiberoptic bronchoscope, the stenotic area was assessed, and a pre-loaded cuffed 3.5 mm ETT was passed through the nose. The subglottic opening was large enough to allow the ETT to pass into the trachea. The tracheotomy tube was removed, and the ETT advanced beyond the tracheal stoma. The cuff was inflated and ventilation confirmed with capnography. A single-stage laryngotracheoplasty with cartilage grafting proceeded uneventfully, and the child was transferred to the pediatric intensive care unit where he remained intubated and sedated for 7 days. Sedation was then discontinued and the child was extubated uneventfully. He returned home after several days of observation.

Decisions as to the type of reconstruction to be performed, the anesthesia to be administered, and use of laryngeal stents after reconstructive surgery have to be individualized to each patient depending on the severity and location of the stenosis. The stent type, length, and placement duration have to be individually tailored. Key factors in successful LTR surgery include close postoperative care and monitoring to minimize complications/morbidities, optimize healing, and ensure timely stent removal, along with subsequent regular periodic surveillance bronchoscopy evaluations for granulation tissue control.

References

1. Myer CM, 3rd, O'Connor DM, Cotton RT. Proposed grading system for subglottic stenosis based on endotracheal tube sizes. *Ann Otol Rhinol Laryngol* 1994; **103**(4 Pt 1): 319–23.

2. Gustafson LM, Hartley BE, Liu JH, *et al.* Single-stage laryngotracheal reconstruction in children: a review of 200 cases. *Otolaryngol Head Neck Surg* 2000; **123**(4): 430–4.

3. Cotton RT, O'Connor DM. Paediatric laryngotracheal reconstruction: 20 years' experience. *Acta Otorhinolaryngol Belg* 1995; **49**(4): 367–72.

4. Zalzal GH. Treatment of laryngotracheal stenosis with anterior and posterior cartilage grafts. A report of 41 children. *Arch Otolaryngol Head Neck Surg* 1993; **119**: 82–6.

5. Cotton RT, Gray SD, Miller RP. Update of the Cincinnati experience in pediatric laryngotracheal reconstruction. *Laryngoscope* 1989; **99**(11): 1111–16.

6. Hartnick CJ, Hartley BE, Lacy PD, *et al.* Surgery for pediatric subglottic stenosis: disease-specific outcomes. *Ann Otol Rhinol Laryngol* 2001; **110**(12): 1109–13.

7. White DR, Cotton RT, Bean JA, Rutter MJ. Pediatric cricotracheal resection: surgical outcomes and risk factor analysis. *Arch Otolaryngol Head Neck Surg* 2005; **131**(10): 896–9.

8. Choi SS, Zalzal GH. Changing trends in neonatal subglottic stenosis. *Otolaryngol Head Neck Surg* 2000; **122**: 61–3.

9. Younis RT, Lazar RH, Astor F. Posterior cartilage graft in single-stage laryngotracheal reconstruction. *Otolaryngol Head Neck Surg* 2003; **129**(3): 168–75.

10. Walner DL, Stern Y, Gerber ME, Rudolph C, Baldwin CY, Cotton RT. Gastroesophageal reflux in patients with subglottic stenosis. *Arch Otolaryngol Head Neck Surg* 1998; **124**(5): 551–5.

11. Maronian NC, Azadeh H, Waugh P, Hillel A. Association of laryngopharyngeal reflux disease and subglottic stenosis. *Ann Otol Rhinol Laryngol* 2001; **110**(7 Pt 1): 606–12.

12. Yellon RF, Parameswaran M, Brandom BW. Decreasing morbidity following laryngotracheal reconstruction in children. *Int J Pediatr Otorhinolaryngol* 1997; **41**(2): 145–54.

13. Halstead LA. Gastroesophageal reflux: A critical factor in pediatric subglottic stenosis. *Otolaryngol Head Neck Surg* 1999; **120**(5): 683–8.

14. Smith LP, Chewaproug L, Spergel JM, Zur KB. Otolaryngologists may not be doing enough to diagnose pediatric eosinophilic esophagitis. *Int J Pediatr Otorhinolaryngol* 2009.

15. Dauer EH, Ponikau JU, Smyrk TC, Murray JA, Thompson DM. Airway manifestations of pediatric eosinophilic esophagitis: a clinical and histopathologic report of an emerging association. *Ann Otol Rhinol Laryngol* 2006; **115**(7): 507–17.

16. Zalzal GH, Choi SS, Patel KM. Ideal timing of pediatric laryngotracheal reconstruction. *Arch Otolaryngol Head Neck Surg* 1997; **123**(2): 206–8.

17. Carr MM, Poje CP, Kingston L, Kielma D, Heard C. Complications in pediatric tracheostomies. *Laryngoscope* 2001; **111**(11 Pt 1): 1925–8.

18. Carron JD, Derkay CS, Strope GL, Nosonchuk JE, Darrow DH. Pediatric tracheotomies: changing indications and outcomes. *Laryngoscope* 2000; **110**(7): 1099–104.

19. Dutton JM, Palmer PM, McCulloch TM, Smith RJ. Mortality in the pediatric patient with tracheotomy. *Head Neck* 1995; **17**(5): 403–8.

20. Eze NN, Wyatt ME, Hartley BE. The role of the anterior cricoid split in facilitating extubation in infants. *Int J Pediatr Otorhinolaryngol* 2005; **69**(6): 843–6.

21. Koppert W, Sittl R, Scheuber K, Alsheimer M, Schmelz M, Schuttler J. Differential modulation of remifentanil-induced analgesia and postinfusion hyperalgesia by S-ketamine and clonidine in humans. *Anesthesiology* 2003; **99**: 152–9.

22. Kissin I, Bright CA, Bradley EL, Jr. The effect of ketamine on opioid-induced acute tolerance: can it explain reduction of opioid consumption with ketamine-opioid analgesic combinations? *Anesth Analg* 2000; **91**(6): 1483–8.

23. De Kock M, Lavand'homme P, Waterloos H. "Balanced analgesia" in the perioperative period: is there a place for ketamine? *Pain* 2001; **92**(3): 373–80.

24. Fu ES, Miguel R, Scharf JE. Preemptive ketamine decreases postoperative narcotic requirements in patients undergoing

abdominal surgery. *Anesth Analg* 1997; **84**(5): 1086–90.

25. Himmelseher S, Durieux ME. Ketamine for perioperative pain management. *Anesthesiology* 2005; **102**: 211–20.

26. Istaphanous GK, Loepke AW. General anesthetics and the developing brain. *Curr Opin Anaesthesiol* 2009; **22**(3): 368–73.

27. Zou X, Patterson TA, Divine RL, *et al.* Prolonged exposure to ketamine increases neurodegeneration in the developing monkey brain. *Int J Dev Neurosci* 2009; **27**(7): 727–31.

28. Koroglu A, Demirbilek S, Teksan H, Sagir O, But AK, Ersoy MO. Sedative, haemodynamic and respiratory effects of dexmedetomidine in children undergoing magnetic resonance imaging examination: preliminary results. *Br J Anaesth* 2005; **94**(6): 821–4.

29. Venn RM, Hell J, Grounds RM. Respiratory effects of dexmedetomidine in the surgical patient requiring intensive care. *Crit Care* 2000; **4**(5): 302–8.

30. Talke P, Lobo E, Brown R. Systemically administered alpha2-agonist-induced peripheral vasoconstriction in humans. *Anesthesiology* 2003; **99**: 65–70.

31. Talke P, Richardson CA, Scheinin M, Fisher DM. Postoperative pharmacokinetics and sympatholytic effects of dexmedetomidine. *Anesth Analg* 1997; **85**(5): 1136–42.

32. Finkel JC, Elrefai A. The use of dexmedetomidine to facilitate opioid and benzodiazepine detoxification in an infant. *Anesth Analg* 2004; **98**(6): 1658–9, table of contents.

33. Wunsch H, Kress JP. A new era for sedation in ICU patients. *JAMA* 2009; **301**(5): 542–4.

34. Bagwell CE. CO2 laser excision of pediatric airway lesions. *J Pediatr Surg* 1990; **25**(11): 1152–6.

35. Werkhaven JA, Weed DT, Ossoff RH. Carbon dioxide laser serial microtrapdoor flap excision of subglottic stenosis. *Arch Otolaryngol Head Neck Surg* 1993; **119**(6): 676–9.

36. Durden F, Sobol SE. Balloon laryngoplasty as a primary treatment for subglottic

stenosis. *Arch Otolaryngol Head Neck Surg* 2007; **133**(8): 772–5.

37. Lee KH, Rutter MJ. Role of balloon dilation in the management of adult idiopathic subglottic stenosis. *Ann Otol Rhinol Laryngol* 2008; **117**(2): 81–4.

38. Cotton RT, Seid AB. Management of the extubation problem in the premature child. Anterior cricoid split as an alternative to tracheotomy. *Ann Otol Rhinol Laryngol* 1980; **89**(6 Pt 1): 508–11.

39. Forte V, Chang MB, Papsin BC. Thyroid ala cartilage reconstruction in neonatal subglottic stenosis as a replacement for the anterior cricoid split. *Int J Pediatr Otorhinolaryngol* 2001; **59**(3): 181–6.

40. White DR, Bravo M, Vijayasekaran S, Rutter MJ, Cotton RT, Elluru RG. Laryngotracheoplasty as an alternative to tracheotomy in infants younger than 6 months. *Arch Otolaryngol Head Neck Surg* 2009; **135**(5): 445–7.

41. Fearon B, Cotton R. Surgical correction of subglottic stenosis of the larynx. Preliminary report of an experimental surgical technique. *Ann Otol Rhinol Laryngol* 1972; **81**(4): 508–13.

42. Jacobs BR, Salman BA, Cotton RT, Lyons K, Brilli RJ. Postoperative management of children after single-stage laryngotracheal reconstruction. *Crit Care Med* 2001; **29**: 164–8.

43. Stern Y, Willging JP, Cotton RT. Use of Montgomery T-tube in laryngotracheal reconstruction in children: is it safe? *Ann Otol Rhinol Laryngol* 1998; **107**(12): 1006–9.

44. Conley JJ. Reconstruction of the subglottic air passage. *Ann Otol Rhinol Laryngol* 1953; **62**(2): 477–95.

45. Monnier P, Savary M, Chapuis G. Partial cricoid resection with primary tracheal anastomosis for subglottic stenosis in infants and children. *Laryngoscope* 1993; **103**(11 Pt 1): 1273–83.

46. Rutter MJ, Hartley BE, Cotton RT. Cricotracheal resection in children. *Arch Otolaryngol Head Neck Surg* 2001; **127**(3): 289–92.

47. Hartley BE, Rutter MJ, Cotton RT. Cricotracheal resection as a primary procedure for laryngotracheal stenosis in children. *Int J Pediatr Otorhinolaryngol* 2000; **54**(2–3): 133–6.

48. Bailey M, Hoeve H, Monnier P. Paediatric laryngotracheal stenosis: a consensus paper from three European centres. *Eur Arch Otorhinolaryngol* 2003; **260**(3): 118–23.

49. Hammer GB. Sedation and analgesia in the pediatric Intensive Care Unit following laryngotracheal reconstruction. *Otolaryngol Clin North Am* 2008; **41**(5): 1023–1044, x–xi.

50. Bauman NM, Oyos TL, Murray DJ, Kao SC, Biavati MJ, Smith RJ. Postoperative care following single-stage laryngotracheoplasty. *Ann Otol Rhinol Laryngol* 1996; **105**(4): 317–22.

51. Rothschild MA, Cotcamp D, Cotton RT. Postoperative medical management in single-stage laryngotracheoplasty. *Arch Otolaryngol Head Neck Surg* 1995; **121**(10): 1175–9.

Chapter

8

Timing of tracheotomy for intubated patients

Alison Wilson, Elias B. Rizk, Kimberly E. Fenton, Thomas K. Lee, and Elizabeth H. Sinz

Case presentation

E.W. is a 67-year-old woman with a medical history of hypertension, obesity, obstructive sleep apnea, diabetes mellitus, and atrial fibrillation. Her social history included a 45 pack-year history of tobacco use and social alcohol consumption. She was admitted to the medical intensive care unit (ICU) for post-hemorrhagic stroke in the right middle cerebral artery territory. The patient was intubated due to poor airway protection, and has failed several attempts to wean completely from ventilator support during the past 2 weeks. The medical intensive care team requested a consult for a tracheotomy 4 days after admission; however, the surgeon consultant was uncomfortable performing the procedure so early after intubation, and asked that further attempts at weaning be tried. After 2 weeks, the patient remains intubated on a low level of ventilator support. Her neurologic function has improved but remains poor. Should this patient undergo a tracheotomy? If so, where should the procedure be performed, in the operating room or in the ICU?

Elective tracheotomy in the intensive care unit

Tracheotomy is one of the oldest known surgical procedures [1], and one of the most common procedures for patients in the ICU [2]. This procedure may be beneficial to the patient for a variety of reasons:

- decrease in dead space ventilation improves ventilation mechanics [3]
- suctioning and bronchial clearance are facilitated
- need for long-term sedation is decreased, reducing associated complications
- access for intermittent mechanical ventilation is available without reintubation
- process of weaning from mechanical ventilation is hastened
- phonation and swallowing are supported [4]
- overall patient comfort is improved.

The development of endotracheal tubes with low-pressure/high-volume cuffs, pushed back the timing of tracheotomy due to concerns that the risk of injury from the procedure had become greater than the risk of prolonged orotracheal intubation. As the potential

Tracheotomy Management: A Multidisciplinary Approach, ed. Peggy A. Seidman,
David Goldenberg and Elizabeth H. Sinz. Published by Cambridge University Press.
© Cambridge University Press 2011.

benefits of earlier tracheotomy have become apparent and the procedure has generally become simpler and arguably safer, earlier tracheotomy has gained popularity.

Some studies have suggested that early tracheotomy may decrease the incidence of pneumonia [5,6], reduce ventilator days, and shorten ICU and overall length of stay [7–10], and even improve survival [11]. Unfortunately, tracheotomy itself may result in various procedural complications if done "early" in a patient's course [12]. This and other studies suggest that early tracheotomy does not improve overall outcome [13–19]. Hence the ongoing debate about the optimal timing of tracheotomy in the intensive care setting continues today [20].

The 1989 American College of Chest Physicians (ACCP) Consensus Conference on Artificial Airways in Patients Receiving Mechanical Ventilation [21] concluded that the appropriate duration of translaryngeal intubation could not be defined. It was suggested that if the anticipated need for mechanical ventilation is longer than 21 days then tracheotomy is preferable to prolonged intubation. For mechanical ventilation anticipated to last between 10 and 21 days, the decision was left to the physician, and daily reassessment was recommended. Since then, numerous efforts have been made to determine which patients, if any, would benefit from early tracheotomy versus those in whom continued weaning would perhaps spare a surgical airway; studies considered not only the outcome for the patient, but also the associated cost. The disparate results between studies reflects many variables: definition of "early" and "late" tracheotomy; primary pathology of the patient population studied; surgical approach and patient's care postprocedure; and outcome variables and how complications of endotracheal tubes and surgical airways are followed-up and measured.

It is unlikely that one approach to timing will be appropriate for all patients who are intubated in the ICU, but there is some evidence that applies to patients with specific illnesses or injuries. Both the condition of the patient before their acute illness as well as the particular illness that led to intubation will play a role in the decision to recommend a tracheotomy. Studies are often retrospective; however, the need for tracheotomy is often a marker for disease severity, making comparisons between patients with and without a tracheotomy uneven. The procedure itself may affect outcomes as a surgical airway may influence the patient's course positively (due to improved ventilator mechanics, comfort, and ease of care) or negatively (due to complications from the procedure itself, bacterial colonization, and transport to and from the ICU). The few prospective studies available are small and typically focus on a limited patient population. In addition, prospective randomized studies of tracheotomy timing reveal that clinicians are not always correct in predicting the need for prolonged ventilation. Therefore, some patients will receive a tracheotomy that they would not need it if they were given more time to wean.

The timing of the tracheotomy procedure must also take into account the clinical status of the patient. The patient with severe hemodynamic instability or requiring extreme ventilator support cannot safely undergo the tracheotomy procedure, although it may be likely they will benefit from the intervention once completed. Furthermore, although some studies indicate that percutaneous tracheotomy may be preferred for certain patient populations, the decision to do the procedure at the bedside versus in the operating room may be due to technical challenges related to patient anatomy. No matter how robust the evidence from studies, the clinician's judgment will still be critical.

Although it is typical for patients to require reduced or no sedation once extubated with a tracheotomy in place, many studies neglect or minimize the importance of patient comfort [22]. Benefits such as ease of care, potential to regain swallowing, ability to participate in physical activities or interact with family and friends, as well as possibility of the patient being able to direct their own care may be more important to patients than to healthcare professionals. The decision about when to perform a tracheotomy should be made after consideration of all these variables in light of the best evidence available from studies of similar patients coupled with thoughtful judgment of the patient's likely outcome and values.

Recommendations based on injury

Spinal cord injury

Acute spinal cord injury (SCI) occurs in the United States at the rate of up to 50 injuries per million persons per year [23]. The average age at the time of SCI is 34, and men are four times more likely than women to be affected. Cervical SCI is a severe injury associated with a high complication rate. Injury at C5 or above is an independent predictor for requirement of mechanical ventilation [24]. Patients with a C2 or C3 lesion will require long-term ventilation and therefore tracheotomy is indicated. As the phrenic nerve innervates the diaphragm via C3, 4, and 5, injuries in this vicinity impair diaphragm function to varying degrees. Injuries at the thoracic level or above also result in loss of intercostal and abdominal muscle function, increasing the risk of atelectasis, pneumonia, and respiratory failure. In general, the frequency of pulmonary complications parallels the degree of respiratory impairment with increasing incidence at progressively higher levels of injury [25].

For those requiring mechanical ventilation, time of intubation is prolonged due to decreased vital capacity, impairment of airway secretion clearance, and high incidence of pneumonia and/or atelectasis [26]. Studies have shown that respiratory complications occur in 50–67% of persons with any SCI [27]. Pneumonia contributes significantly to complications in patients with low cervical SCIs occurring in 50–75% of those with complete lesions and up to 50% with incomplete lesions [23,28].

Harrop et al. found a strong relationship between tracheotomy and patient age greater than 45, pre-existing medical conditions, pre-morbid lung disease, and presence of pneumonia [28]. Hassid et al. found that in patients with a C5–T1 injury, 68% had respiratory failure requiring intubation. This included patients with complete and incomplete SCIs, though need for intubation was more prevalent in those with complete injuries (91% versus 38%). It is notable that in patients with incomplete spine injuries requiring intubation at any point, 50% ultimately required a tracheotomy [23]. Patients with a low cervical or high thoracic injury are often not intubated until several days after admission. This is because their diaphragmatic function is adequate for oxygenation and ventilation, but the loss of intercostal function prevents normal coughing and sighing, which is necessary for clearance of secretions and atelectasis. Their swallowing is also frequently affected so that aspiration is more likely. These patients require frequent reassessment of their airway and respiratory status during the first week after injury. Evidence of deterioration should be addressed swiftly and aggressively to avoid catastrophic results [23].

The timing of tracheotomy for patients with low cervical and high thoracic cord injury is not consistent. In a retrospective study that evaluated the benefits and safety of early versus late tracheotomy in patients with traumatic SCI requiring mechanical ventilation, Romero et al. [29] defined early tracheotomy as a procedure performed during days 0–7 after intubation and late tracheotomy performed after day 7. In this study, early tracheotomy was associated with decreased time of mechanical ventilation, reduced ICU stay, lower overall complication rate, and trend toward decreased mortality. However, there was no significant difference between groups in the number of patients who suffered pneumonia, both pre- and post-tracheotomy. The number of complications such as bleeding, stoma infection, suture dehiscence, granuloma, and concentric tracheal stenosis was higher in the late tracheotomy group. While some cite concerns for an increased infection risk after spine stabilization with early tracheotomy, no difference was noted between the groups [29].

Spinal cord injury: summary

Spinal cord lesions are associated with a high incidence of severe respiratory failure and pneumonia, with increased risk generally corresponding to a higher level of injury. The majority of patients who require intubation will require a tracheotomy. In recent years, early tracheotomy has become the most commonly recommended strategy for patients with respiratory failure due to SCI because of its low morbidity and mortality. When performed before day 7, early tracheotomy can decrease duration of mechanical ventilation and ICU length of stay, potentially allowing the patient to proceed to rehabilitation earlier.

Traumatic brain injury

It is expected that the sickest patients will require the longest time on a ventilator [21], which is best exemplified in patients with a neurologic insult. Patients with a head injury are at an increased risk of undergoing tracheotomy due to the prolonged need for mechanical ventilation [30]. While indications for intubation in severe traumatic brain injury (TBI) are generally well established, current care algorithms come up short when predicting the best time to employ tracheotomy in this setting [31–33].

Outcome measures that have been studied include traditional ones such as overall clinical outcome and hospital or ICU length of stay, as well as more respiratory-specific measures such as incidence of laryngeal damage, degree of improvement in respiratory mechanics, rate of ventilator-associated pneumonia (VAP), and ease of care [34].

Early tracheotomy has been compared with late tracheotomy both retrospectively and in some relatively small prospective series [35–37], which suggest a higher incidence of positive outcomes in patients with tracheotomy. Other studies have not found a favorable influence from tracheotomy [5,36–39]. Some studies noted improvement in length of stay parameters but no change in mortality or pneumonia rates [37,40–43].

Bouderka et al. performed a randomized, prospective trial of 62 patients with severe TBI with tracheotomy at 5 days versus prolonged endotracheal intubation. Early tracheotomy decreased both total days of mechanical ventilation, and mechanical ventilation time after the development of pneumonia [31]. However, they found no difference in overall rates of pneumonia and mortality between the two groups.

On the other hand, a small prospective study, found fewer intubation-associated complications and improved mortality in patients receiving early tracheotomy as compared with prolonged mechanical ventilation [44]. However, there has been some support for decreased rates of pneumonia with early (less than day 7) tracheotomy [10].

The multicenter-controlled trial by Sugerman et al. randomized 112 selected patients into early (days 3–5) and late (days 10–14) tracheotomy. In the subset of patients with TBI, the authors did not find any difference in the incidence of pneumonia, ICU length of stay, or death when comparing early or late tracheotomy groups with continued intubation. However, the ICU length of stay among tracheotomized patients is shorter in the early surgery group than in the late tracheotomy group (20 ± 2 versus 38 ± 5 days, $P = 0.0008$) [45]. Functional outcome has not been well studied.

If there is a benefit to early tracheotomy, it would follow that identifying factors early during admission to maximize this opportunity would be useful. Glasgow coma scores (GCS) less than 8 is the most prominent patient characteristic that supports early tracheotomy [7,31,37,46,47]. Qureshi suggests that an infratentorial lesion or injury is highly correlated with need for tracheotomy [48]. Another report found a 100% tracheotomy rate in patients with craniotomy and age greater than 50, craniotomy, intracranial pressure (ICP) monitor and age greater than 40, and craniotomy and GCS less than 4 at 24 hours [30]. These studies all indicate that the severity of brain injury correlates with the potential benefit of early tracheotomy. In contrast, some patients with severe brain injury are candidates for extubation, despite failure to meet customary extubation criteria. Furthermore, the potential for survival must be considered in patients with severe brain injuries before a tracheotomy is recommended. Patients who are likely to progress to brain death or who will be rapidly moved to palliative care only are not likely to benefit from tracheotomy.

When deciding the timing of the procedure, an additional consideration regarding early tracheotomy in patients with severe brain injury is the effect of the stimulus on the patient's ICP. If the ICP is very labile or sensitive, adequate anesthesia and monitoring must be assured while performing the procedure to avoid a significant elevation in ICP. This may affect location, approach, or timing of the procedure. None of the studies reviewed evaluated these particular issues regarding tracheotomy and TBI.

Traumatic brain injury: summary

If GCS is less than 8, early tracheotomy (before day 7) can reduce the duration of mechanical ventilation and ICU length of stay. There is conflicting evidence regarding the effect of early tracheotomy on the incidence of pneumonia. There is no convincing evidence that early tracheotomy modifies mortality, airway injury, or hospital length of stay. A prospective randomized trial may further define and clarify the role of tracheotomy timing in patients with brain injuries. However, it would be useful if such a study included outcome measures of functional status and would focus on patients with a relatively high chance of survival.

Tracheotomy for traumatic injuries that do not include the central nervous system

Some trauma patient populations are very straightforward, such as the patient with severe laryngeal trauma where it is clear tracheotomy should be performed immediately. However, patients with non-central nervous system trauma may be one of the most difficult to predict the definitive need and timing for tracheotomy.

Multiple studies have evaluated critical care patients in the absence of concurrent brain injury and early versus late tracheotomy. Lesnik et al. evaluated tracheotomy (before or after 4 days) and noted decreased duration of mechanical ventilation and decreased incidence of pneumonia [49]. Another retrospective study evaluated tracheotomy before 3 days or after 7 days and found a decrease in the incidence of pneumonia [5]. Retrospective and prospective trials have shown a decrease in duration of mechanical ventilation, and a decrease in ICU and hospital length of stay, and hospital charges [10,40,50]. Some have looked at the probability of survival and acuity via the Injury Severity Score. They found benefit in early tracheotomy in those patients requiring mechanical ventilation with a greater than 25% probability of survival [51]. Others have identified particular injury patterns and combinations shown to have a high (> 90%) chance of needing a tracheotomy and recommend early intervention if these risk factors are identified [30]. Patients with severe chest wall injuries, including flail chest and/or multiple rib fractures may require prolonged mechanical ventilation, although some do not, particularly if excellent pain control can be provided early with continuous thoracic epidural analgesia [52,53]. In addition, the pre-injury health and nutrition status of the patient plays an important role in their ability to recover from a traumatic injury. There is also some evidence that burn patients may not benefit from early tracheotomy [54].

A consensus paper was published by the EAST Practice Management Guidelines Work Group in 2009 and found good evidence that there is no mortality difference between early tracheotomy, late tracheotomy, or prolonged intubation. There was some evidence that early tracheotomy may decrease the length of stay and duration of mechanical ventilation for trauma patients without head injury and may also decrease the rate of pneumonia in trauma patients [55].

Multiple trauma: summary

Current guidelines endorse considerations of early tracheotomy for all trauma patients anticipated to require mechanical ventilation for more than 7 days.

Use of tracheotomy in craniomaxillofacial trauma

General indications for performing tracheotomy after maxillofacial injury include upper airway obstruction, facial edema, insecure orotracheal or nasotracheal intubation, airway diversion during and after facial fracture repair, need for tracheobronchial hygiene, and long-term ventilation [56]. There are some, however, who advocate persistent nasotracheal intubation or airway diversion procedures such as submental intubation. Specific patient variables that have been shown to be predictive of the need for long-term ventilation include head injury, GCS, mechanism of injury, facial injury pattern, and patient comorbidities [57]. Tracheotomy was a first choice for patients with panfacial fractures or those with loss of consciousness and midfacial fractures [58].

Facial fractures are the major type of maxillofacial trauma and result in airway compromise due to posterior displacement of midface structures into the oropharynx or due to severe hemorrhage and edema in the surrounding areas. Some unique advantages of tracheotomy in managing facial fractures include facilitating the placement of maxillomandibular fixation and clearing the nasal and oral passages of any artificial tubes. Ng *et al.* found that one-third (of a total of 64) of patients with midface fractures required intubation [59]. A survey of anesthesiologists and surgeons showed that tracheotomy was used in 11.6% of patients with mandibular, panfacial, and Le Fort fractures [58]. In addition, 43.5% of patients with Le Fort III fractures needed tracheotomy compared with 9.1% in patients with Le Fort I and II fractures [60]. A study by Thompson *et al.* confirmed that patients with Le Fort III fractures are at greater risk for airway compromise; 26.5% of patients with Le Fort fractures had airway compromise and 33.3% needed a tracheotomy [61].

In a retrospective study at a level 1 trauma center, tracheotomy was most commonly performed in patients with high-velocity injuries resulting in comminuted mandibular and midface fractures. The timing of facial fracture repair was adjusted to coincide with the patient's medical stability and need for tracheotomy to facilitate pulmonary toilet. Patients receiving mechanical ventilation typically have severe head injury and/or pulmonary contusion in which early tracheotomy was deemed beneficial from a clinical point of view [56].

Facial trauma: summary

Depending on the nature of the trauma, tracheotomy may be the primary method of securing the airway, particularly if upper airway anatomy is so distorted that nasotracheal or laryngo-tracheal intubation is impossible. The need for conversion of a laryngotracheal tube to a tracheotomy depends upon the type of facial fracture sustained by the patient, combined with comorbidities such as severe neurologic or pulmonary injury. Nasotracheal, orotra-cheal, or transtracheal options are most common; however, submental and submandibular approaches offer an interesting alternative. The method of intubation chosen will depend on each patient's situation and expertise of the trauma team.

Role of tracheotomy in cardiac surgery patients

Developments in technology and pharmacology and better understanding of cardiac patho-physiology have led to the continued expansion of procedures available to patients of all ages with cardiac diseases. A wide spectrum of procedures is offered to patients that are older and sicker and with a wider spectrum of non-cardiac, multisystem comorbidity. Airway and pulmonary complications are among many seen in a patient after cardiac surgery. Poor preoperative pulmonary status along with use of narcotic analgesics for control of chest pain after surgery have been implicated as causes of postoperative pulmonary dysfunction. Greater pain intensity is linked to increased frequency of atelectasis. Furthermore, physiological derangements such as fluid imbalance, immobility, ineffective cough pattern, and decreased mucociliary clearance put the patient at risk for pulmonary complications.

Prolonged ventilator support is seen in a small percentage of cardiac surgery patients who experience respiratory complications, such as pneumonia with subsequent respiratory failure, adult respiratory distress syndrome, and cerebrovascular accidents that decrease the patient's ability to protect and maintain their airway. Morbidity after open-heart surgery from prolonged ventilator support (> 72 h) was first studied by LoCicero *et al.* in a cohort of 581 patients. Of 9.9% of patients that required mechanical ventilation past 72 h, the overall mortality was 43%. Among the survivors, 45% received a tracheotomy at about postoperative day 14. Of these, 26% were eventually extubated, 37% required a chronic tracheotomy, and 37% died. The complication rate for patients with orotracheal intubation was 65% compared with 37% for those with tracheotomy; however, the rate of serious complications was higher with tracheotomy. No patients in this cohort died as a direct result of airway management [62].

Timing

The performance of earlier tracheotomy when extubation is not foreseen within a few days of the operation is supported by the literature and has been associated with a favorable outcome on mortality rate and overall infection rate in critically ill patients. A large retrospective study analyzed the effect of timing and technique of tracheotomy on mortality and morbidity in cardiovascular surgery patients. Yavas *et al.* concluded that both percutaneous and surgical tracheotomy procedures are safe, although the rate of significant complications was 6.3% (13 of 205). There was a statistically and clinically significant decrease in mortality between patients who underwent early (≤ 7 days) versus late (> 7 days) tracheotomy. In this cohort, there was no statistically significant difference in preoperative risk factors, primary operation, tracheotomy timing, and number of tracheotomy-related complication rates between the open surgical and percutaneous technique [11].

ICU length of stay and mechanical ventilation time are generally shorter for cardiovascular surgery patients who received earlier tracheotomies (< 7 days) versus later. The postoperative infection rate was lower, and patient cooperation, postoperative mobilization, and oral feeding rates are higher in the early tracheotomy group [11,63].

Is tracheotomy a risk factor for mediastinitis after median sternotomy?

A commonly held belief is that tracheotomy, in particular early tracheotomy, increases the risk of mediastinitis in patients who have had median sternotomies. The purported mechanism is spread of bacteria from the tracheotomy into the wound. Standard thoracic surgery texts advise placing the stoma as far away from a median sternotomy as possible, to avoid risk of mediastinitis [64]. Some literature even recommends using bilateral incisions for coronary artery bypass grafting instead of median sternotomy in patients with a tracheotomy in situ preoperatively [65].

However, the risk of mediastinitis after tracheotomy in post-median sternotomy cardiac patients is actually low. Although there is evidence of superficial sternal wound bacterial colonization similar to bacteria cultured from the tracheotomy wound, Stamenkovic found no evidence of related mediastinitis [66]. To evaluate the incidence of mediastinitis related to tracheotomy, Gaudino *et al.* conducted a retrospective analysis of a series of 5095 consecutive patients who underwent early tracheotomy after cardiac surgery [63]. Baseline demographic prevalence of diabetes mellitus, coronary artery bypass time, total operative time, and rate of use of internal thoracic artery for coronary bypass were not statistically different between patients who received tracheotomy versus those who did not. Nonetheless, the rate of chronic pulmonary disease was much higher in the group that required tracheotomy. Similarly, duration of ICU stay and mechanical ventilation and incidence of sepsis and renal failure and operative and follow-up mortality rates were significantly higher among patients who had tracheotomy. These findings emphasize the compromised general condition of these patients.

Despite the added risk factors for deep sternal wound infection, none of the patients who received tracheotomy developed postoperative mediastinitis. There was no correlation between the time from operation to performance of tracheotomy and incidence of microbiological positivity of the sternal wound. There was no similarity in bacterial isolates between wound cultures in patients with dehiscent subcutaneous tissue at the sternotomy site and cultures from bronchial secretions. This argues strongly against an association between a tracheotomy cannula and spread of infection to the median sternotomy site [63].

Studies show that concern for peritracheotomy infection, mediastinitis, and sternal wound infections appears unsubstantiated after percutaneous dilatational tracheotomy in this patient cohort [63,67]. These authors speculate that the small skin incision and minimal disruption of tissue planes required for percutaneous dilatational tracheotomy reduce the risk of peritracheotomy infection. Westphal *et al.* [68] and Stamenkovic *et al.* [66] also report no chest wound infection associated with percutaneous dilatational tracheotomy. Bacchetta and colleagues conducted a retrospective study to compare open versus bedside percutaneous dilatational tracheotomy and there was no significant difference in wound infection or mediastinitis in both patient groups [67].

Taken together, the results from various studies reject the hypothesis that infection may easily spread from the tracheotomy to the sternal wound despite the tracheotomy being performed soon after cardiac surgery. In addition, they support the idea that there is no clinically significant link between early postoperative tracheotomy and mediastinitis in patients after median sternotomy.

Technique

Frequently reported complications from tracheotomy in critically ill patients are oxygen desaturation, bleeding, aspiration, and wound infection. Impairment of gas exchange and oxygen desaturation are considered the most dangerous complications. Westphal and colleagues [68] conducted a prospective study of 120 cardiac surgery patients who had conventional open, minimally invasive percutaneous dilatational or translaryngeal tracheotomy technique. The main areas of investigation included oxygenation index, complications, infections, and cost. This study indicated that, with all three tracheotomy procedures, there was an initial decrease in oxygenation index, but the decrease was significantly less with the minimally invasive techniques. This may be important in cardiac surgery patients who have a history of smoking or a diagnosis of chronic obstructive pulmonary disease. In patients with respiratory insufficiency, such as adult respiratory distress syndrome or sepsis, a prolonged and severe decrease of oxygenation index increases the risk of tissue hypoxia. Likewise, even mild hypoxia can highly impair cardiac function in patients that have coronary insufficiency or cardiac valve malfunction. Therefore, the authors recommend a minimally invasive tracheotomy technique for such patients, except those with a baseline oxygenation index of less than 100 to avoid hypoxia and associated morbidity during the procedure.

Any tracheotomy procedure poses the problem of wound contamination by bacteria. The incidence of bacterial wound contamination appears to be lower with a minimally invasive technique than with the conventional method [69,70]. One of the initial studies done by Stauffer and colleagues [12] looked at 150 critically ill adult patients investigating the complications and consequences of open versus minimally invasive tracheotomy. In open tracheotomy, the incidence of wound contamination was as high as 36%. In a later study, Westphal and colleagues [68] noted a 35% incidence of wound contamination after open tracheotomy, despite all procedures being performed under aseptic conditions.

More interestingly, the spectrum of bacterial culture found within the wound was almost identical to that found on tracheal and bronchial probes of the same patients. It seemed like open tracheotomy resulted in contamination of the wound with patients' own tracheal and bronchial bacteria. Patients that had minimally invasive techniques who were checked routinely for bacterial colonization did not show any wound infection or irritation [67].

Cardiac surgery patients: summary

The addition of tracheotomy to almost any diagnosis-related group is viewed as a surrogate for the severity of illness. There is some evidence for decreased mortality in cardiac surgery patients who undergo early tracheotomy (≤ 7 days) if they cannot be weaned from mechanical ventilation in the first few days after surgery. Other important benefits of tracheotomy include simplified nursing care, improved pulmonary toilet, reduced occurrence of pneumonia, and expedited ventilatory weaning [71]. The improved patient comfort reduces the need for sedation and allows the patient to participate in their care, rehabilitation, and decision-making. More rapid weaning may result in earlier transfer from the ICU and thus cost savings. A percutaneous technique is advocated.

Tracheotomies in elderly and chronically ill patients

The number of tracheotomies performed on elderly and chronically ill patients due to ongoing respiratory failure has increased considerably in recent years, possibly due to the success of critical care treatment. At present, tracheotomy is a common airway management plan for patients with respiratory failure or airway management issues lasting beyond 7–14 days [55].

The placement of tracheotomy in elderly, critically ill patients may result in significant impairments in swallowing. Cognitive decline associated with dementia and Alzheimer's disease, conditions more common in old age, may also interfere with the functional aspect of swallowing [72]. These effects may affect the nutrition and hydration of already frail and medically compromised patients.

The possibility of accidental decannulation is compounded in the elderly who may have a decreased cognitive ability secondary to prolonged illness, polypharmacy, and unfamiliar surroundings, increasing the incidence of confusion and delirium [73]. Elderly patients are also at risk of developing psychosocial and psychological distress due to placement of a tracheotomy. There is also the anxiety associated with tube change and possible limited understanding related to difficulty processing new information [74].

The incidence of respiratory infection is also increased due to interference with the body's normal host defenses and promotion of lower airway colonization with nosocomial pathogens most likely originating from aspiration of oropharyngeal secretions [75]. The elderly are more likely to have tracheotomies longer than younger patients. Good clinical care can significantly reduce risks and improve the chances of not requiring the reinstitution of mechanical ventilation.

Ventilator associated pneumonia (VAP) is a common problem in patients on long-term mechanical ventilation in the ICU. Chastre and Fagon reported an incidence estimated between 8% and 28% of intubated patients and mortality between 25% and 50% [76]. Some data indicated that repeated intubations and movements out of the ICU for the procedure were associated with an increased incidence of VAP [77]. However, in an historical cohort study of patients 65 years or older that underwent a tracheotomy from March 2003 to January 2007, Schneider *et al.* documented no increase in the incidence of VAP for patients taken to the operating room for their tracheotomy. Based on this an operating room-based tracheotomy should not be delayed for fear of causing VAP in an elderly patient. This study also confirms that an early tracheotomy (< 7 days) leads to a decrease in total admission time and ICU admission time [78]. In addition, the earlier tracheotomy group had a lower rate of VAP despite a higher average number of intubations. There was a trend, but no significant difference, towards lower mortality in the early tracheotomy group. In many cases, the placement of tracheotomy enabled the patient to be moved out of the ICU to a ventilator step-down unit, which may be an important consideration for efficient use of hospital resources.

The ideal timing of tracheotomy is still a significant question for intensivists. Future prospective studies should look at the outcomes in critically ill geriatric patients who are given tracheotomies within 7 days of continuous mechanical ventilation to determine if these patients benefit (e.g., incidence of VAP, total admission time, and mortality) as suggested by retrospective data [6,77].

Elderly patients requiring tracheotomy after prolonged mechanical ventilation cannot be assured of prolonged survival. The need for tracheotomy in an elderly patient is a marker for poor outcome. In a study by Baskin *et al.*, of 78 tracheotomy patients over 65 years of age, 56% died in the hospital, 44% were discharged, and 77% received a gastrostomy tube [79].

The usual goals of tracheotomy are often not realized in the elderly critically ill population. In most patients, tracheotomy does not lead to ventilator independence. In patients with reduced mental status not much benefit is derived from tracheotomy due to reduced sensory input. Some patients find it hard to speak or swallow after the procedure and require a gastrostomy tube almost at the same time as the tracheotomy. The cost benefit is only seen in facilities that allow ventilator-dependent patients with tracheotomies to be transferred to a lower monitored setting [79].

Given the aforementioned considerations, elderly and severely ill patients with respiratory failure derive questionable benefits from tracheotomy. The intangible benefits, such as proper oral care and comfort, and ease of family members to see the patient have an oral tube converted to a tracheotomy are recognized. However, it is unrealistic to give hope to the patient and family that tracheotomy in a critically ill elderly patient with prolonged mechanical ventilation can prolong life.

A closer look should be taken at whether tracheotomy is prolonging life or extending dying or suffering in the critically ill elderly patient.

Optimizing post-tracheotomy care and management

Tracheotomy teams have been implemented in a small number of hospitals in Australia and overseas resulting in reported beneficial outcomes. The development of the team brought together clinical nurse consultant, physiotherapist, speech pathologist, dietician, social worker, and medical officers. Intensive care workers and respiratory therapy specialists provide a consultant service as required [58].

For patients over 65, a clinical nurse specialist for older person acute care is also included in the team to assess and manage special needs and with the view to prevent complications and smooth transition to discharge and beyond when the tracheotomy is likely to be long term. Referral to a gerontologist is made when required. The team meets weekly to conduct ward rounds and consult on every inpatient with a tracheotomy, and feed back to the treating team with advice regarding tracheotomy care and progress. This team pilot model has shown that benefits of a multidisciplinary approach to tracheotomy management are amplified for older people by including consideration of age-related physiology together with psychological and social issues that significantly impact on clinical outcomes [59].

Elderly and chronically ill patients: summary

The decision to do tracheotomy based solely on duration of mechanical ventilation is conceptualized too narrowly. In the elderly or chronically ill patient the criteria for determining the appropriateness of tracheotomy requires a realistic appraisal of overall outcome. Failure to consider the complex needs and increased risks associated with advanced age and comorbidities can lead to unnecessary or unwanted procedures in this group.

Indications for tracheotomy in pediatrics

The indications for performing a tracheotomy in the child while multifactorial fall into three major categories: airway anomalies, need for chronic ventilation, and facilitation of pulmonary toilet (see Table 8.1) [80–82].

Table 8.1 Indications for tracheotomy

Airway anomalies

Congenital
Craniofacial abnormalities
Laryngomalacia
Subglottic stenosis
Subglottic web
Tracheomalacia
Vocal cord paralysis

Acquired
Anaphylaxis
Inhalation injuries from corrosives or smoke
Infections
 Croup
 Epiglottitis
 Laryngopapillomatosis
 Subglottic stenosis

Trauma to head or neck
Tumors of airway or neck
 Cystic hygroma
 Hemangioma
Vocal cord paralysis

Need for chronic ventilation and/or facilitation of pulmonary toilet

Central nervous system disease
Central apnea or hypoventilation
Chronic lung disease
Coma
Neuromuscular disease
Unconscious state
Diaphragmatic dysfunction
Prematurity
Sleep disorders

Timing of tracheotomy in pediatrics

Timing of tracheotomy appears to be variable; although related to the severity of illness, and there are no guidelines or standards of care in children. The decision to perform a tracheotomy is multifactorial and is influenced not only by the needs of the patient but also by the beliefs of the healthcare team as well as the needs of the family. While some may consider this procedure as simple with many potential benefits, others may regard it as disfiguring and stigmatizing.

In children, there have been only a few retrospective studies that examine the timing of tracheotomy. Graf and colleagues recently characterized patients undergoing tracheotomy in a large, academic children's hospital [80]. The authors describe three groups of patients undergoing tracheotomy in a mixed medical-surgical pediatric ICU: prolonged mechanical ventilation; elective tracheotomy; and emergent tracheotomy. Their data suggest that hospital length of stay is longest in patients that have prolonged courses of mechanical ventilation. The study also reports similar discharge times from the ICU once a tracheotomy is performed in all three groups. Once a tracheotomy is performed, patients undergoing prolonged mechanical ventilation may be rapidly weaned or stabilized on chronic ventilation and discharged from the ICU at the same postoperative interval as patients undergoing elective or emergent tracheotomy. In their study, the short-term follow-up revealed a mortality rate of 13%, with no deaths related to the tracheotomy. The authors did not report on short-term complication rates associated with tracheotomy.

The prolonged mechanical ventilation group also incurred significantly higher mean costs as compared with the elective and emergent tracheotomy groups ($267 892 versus $79 395 and $139 850).

The biases of the healthcare team impacting on the decision to perform a tracheotomy in pediatric patients were recently studied in a survey distributed to pediatric critical care physicians from 16 different institutions in Canada [82]. The investigators found there was a low incidence in use of tracheotomy in the general pediatric critical care population (< 1.5%) and that 51% of respondents agree that tracheotomy is underused in children. Nearly 60% of respondents also agreed that tracheotomy reduces the risk of VAP and ventilator days and improves patient comfort. However, 59% of respondents perceive that tracheotomy is an aggressive procedure and 81% believe that risks associated with the procedure outweigh potential benefits. Taira et al. distributed an anonymous web-based study to members of four national professional societies with the goal of further studying beliefs surrounding timing of tracheotomy [83]. Preliminary results indicate that the majority of practitioners do not believe that adult guidelines apply to children, nor is there a consensus as to the optimal timing of tracheotomy in critically injured children. Furthermore, most practitioners believe that children can be ventilated safely for longer than adults.

Despite the studies mentioned above, there is little evaluation of the medical benefits of earlier tracheotomy in the pediatric population. An anonymous web-based study by Fenton et al. indicates that the majority of practitioners do not believe that adult guidelines apply to children [83]. For pediatric intensivists and surgeons to take a uniform approach toward the timing of tracheotomy, more well-designed studies are necessary.

Timing of tracheotomy in pediatric trauma

Injury is the leading cause of death in children accounting for more than 15 000 deaths annually. Injuries are also a leading cause of hospitalization and pose a serious economic burden. Almost one-quarter of all children injured in the United States each year require medical attention, resulting in 17 billion dollars in medical costs [84]. Pediatric trauma patients often have prolonged hospitalizations with secondary in-hospital morbidities. Early rehabilitation is fundamental in improving outcome. Many patients, especially those with severe neurologic injury, require tracheotomy to facilitate airway protection and secretion clearance. Unlike the adult trauma literature, in which guidelines advocate for early placement of tracheotomy (defined as tracheotomy within first 7 days of hospitalization) [55], there are no practice guidelines in children. Timing of the tracheotomy appears to be variable due to concerns for complications and both short- and long-term risks.

There have been no prospective randomized studies to examine the timing of tracheotomy in the pediatric trauma patient. In a retrospective study, Palmieri et al. described the benefits of early tracheotomy in severely burned children, many of whom had inhalation injuries [81]. In their study 38 children underwent tracheotomy on average of 3.9 days after hospital admission and they reported improved lung compliance post-procedure. There was no comparison group so no other benefits were described. Their complication rate was low and there were no deaths in their population.

Preliminary data by Fenton *et al.* characterize pediatric trauma patients undergoing tracheotomy, using a regional trauma database of over 3300 patients that was reviewed over 11 years [85]. Very few patients who were mechanically ventilated for more than 5 days underwent a tracheotomy (0.9% of the total trauma population). In their study population, pediatric patients undergoing tracheotomy were more severely injured (higher injury severity scores) and lower GCS than patients without tracheotomies. The tracheotomy group had higher rates of nosocomial complications, including increased incidence of pneumonia (50% versus 18.6%), decubitus ulcers (22.2% versus 4.7%), and sepsis (26.7%), and were less likely to be discharged home (3.3% versus 24.4%) compared with patients that did not undergo tracheotomy. The authors adjusted for severity of injury and the rates of all complications (pneumonia, decubitus ulcers, and sepsis) remained higher for those with tracheotomies.

In preliminary work by Taira *et al.*, the timing of tracheotomy was studied retrospectively in a larger pediatric trauma population using the National Trauma Data Bank (NTDB) (NTDB® version 6.2 is a national registry of hospital admissions maintained by the American College of Surgeons) [86,87]. Seven hundred trauma facilities nationwide contributed to the NTDB from 2001 to 2005. There were a total of 1 191 215 patients included in the NTDB; 4502 (7.1%) were pediatric patients of whom 159 underwent non-emergent tracheotomy. One-third (54 of 159) underwent early (≤ 7 days) tracheotomy with a mean age of 9.5 years and 61% were male. Early tracheotomy was associated with a lower rate of pneumonia (5.6% versus 23.8%), shorter than average ventilator days (11.2 versus 26.1), shorter than average ICU length of stay (16.4 versus 36.6), and hospital length of stay (29.9 versus 44.5). Mortality rates were similar (5.6% versus 3.8%). Adjusting for major risk factors of illness severity, ventilator days, and ICU and hospital length of stay all remained statistically significant using multivariate analysis. Although the study has all the limitations of an investigation done from an administrative database, it is one of the first that demonstrates potential benefit of early tracheotomy in pediatric trauma patients. Benefits of early tracheotomy may have been seen in this study as opposed to the study by Fenton because of a larger tracheotomy population and multi-institution practices as opposed to a single institution practice.

Pediatric patients: summary

The optimal timing for performing tracheotomy in critically injured children remains controversial and unknown. Although this question is actively being studied, further multi-institution studies are needed to develop evidence-based guidelines for tracheotomy placement and timing in pediatric trauma patients.

Conclusions

The patient presented at the start of the chapter continued to have a poor neurologic response and her family was asked what they believed she would want to do if able to decide for herself. It was explained that she could remain intubated and on the ventilator, she could undergo a tracheotomy procedure and would likely be weaned from the ventilator at least part of the time. This intervention would also allow her to leave the ICU and go to a rehabilitation facility or nursing home. A third option was offered despite her inadequate weaning parameters (i.e., removing the endotracheal tube). It was explained that if she developed respiratory distress, either she could be reintubated, and a tracheotomy would then be recommended, or she could be given medications to keep her comfortable. The family expressed that the patient had been unwell for many years and did not want to be confined to a nursing home. The facility liaison indicated that she would not meet criteria for inpatient rehabilitation. The decision was made to extubate her with a plan not to reintubate her if she became dyspneic. She was able to breathe comfortably, and was eventually discharged to a hospice facility.

References

1. Fischler L, Erhart S, Kleger GR, Frutiger A. Prevalence of tracheotomy in ICU patients: a nation-wide survey in Switzerland. *Intensive Care Med* 2000; **26**(10): 1428–33.

2. Rana S, Pendem S, Pogodzinski MS, Hubmayr RD, Gajic O. Tracheotomy in critically ill patients. *Mayo Clin Proc* 2005; **80**(12): 1632–8.

3. Davis K Jr, Campbell RS, Johannigman JA, Valente JF, Branson RD. Changes in respiratory mechanics after tracheostomy. *Arch Surg* 1999; **134**: 59–62.

4. Jaeger JM, Littlewood KA, Durbin CG Jr. The role of tracheotomy in weaning from mechanical ventilation. *Respir Care* 2002; **47**(4): 469–80; discussion 81–2.

5. Kluger Y, Paul DB, Lucke J, *et al*. Early tracheotomy in trauma patients. *Eur J Emerg Med* 1996; **3**(2): 95–101.

6. Rumbak MJ, Newton M, Truncale T, *et al*. A prospective, randomized, study comparing early percutaneous dilational tracheotomy to prolonged translaryngeal intubation (delayed tracheotomy) in critically ill medical patients. *Crit Care Med* 2004; **32**(8): 1689–94.

7. Teoh WH, Goh KY, Chan C. The role of early tracheotomy in critically ill neurosurgical patients. *Ann Acad Med Singapore* 2001; **30**(3): 234–8.

8. Lesnik Teoh WH, Goh KY, Chan C. The role of early tracheotomy in critically ill neurosurgical patients. *Ann Acad Med Singapore* 2001; **30**(3): 234–8.

9. Koh WY, Lew TW, Chin NM, Wong MF. Tracheotomy in a neuro-intensive care setting: indications and timing. *Anaesth Intensive Care* 1997; **25**(4): 365–8.

10. Rodriguez JL, Steinberg SM, Luchetti FA, *et al*. Early tracheotomy for primary airway management in the surgical critical care setting. *Surgery* 1990; **108**(4): 655–9.

11. Yavas S, Yagar S, Mavioglu L, *et al*. Tracheostomy: how and when should it be done in cardiovascular surgery ICU? *J Card Surg* 2009; **24**: 11–18.

12. Stauffer JL, Olson DE, Petty TL. Complications and consequences of endotracheal intubation and tracheotomy. A prospective study of 150 critically ill adult patients. *Am J Med* 1981; **70**: 65–76.

13. Dunham CM, LaMonica C. Prolonged tracheal intubation in the trauma patient. *J Trauma* 1984; **24**(2): 120–4.

14. Arola MK. Tracheotomy and its complications. A retrospective study of 794 tracheostomized patients. *Ann Chir Gynaecol* 1981; **70**(3): 96–106.

15. Gaudet PT, Peerless A, Sasaki CT, Kirchner JA. Pediatric tracheotomy and associated complications. *Laryngoscope* 1978; **88**(10): 1633–41.

16. Kapadia FN, Bajan KB, Raje KV. Airway accidents in intubated intensive care unit patients: an epidemiological study. *Crit Care Med* 2000; **28**(3): 659–64.

17. Bryant LR, Trinkle JK, Mobin-Uddin K, Baker J, Griffen WO Jr. Bacterial colonization profile with tracheal intubation and mechanical ventilation. *Arch Surg* 1972; **104**(5): 647–51.

18. El-Naggar M, Sadagopan S, Levine H, Kantor H, Collins VJ. Factors influencing choice between tracheotomy and prolonged translaryngeal intubation in acute respiratory failure: a prospective study. *Anesth Analg* 1976; **55**(2): 195–201.

19. Maziak DE, Meade MO, Todd TR. The timing of tracheotomy: a systematic review. *Chest* 1998; **114**(2): 605–9.

20. Durbin CG Jr. Indications for and timing of tracheotomy. *Respir Care* 2005; **50**(4): 483–7.

21. Plummer AL, Gracey DR. Consensus conference on artificial airways in patients receiving mechanical ventilation. *Chest* 1989; **96**: 178–80.

22. Blot F, Similowski T, Trouillet Chardon J, *et al.* Early tracheotomy versus prolonged endotracheal intubation in unselected severely ill ICU patients. *Intensive Care Med* 2008; **34**: 1779–87.

23. Hassid VJ, Schinco MA, Tepas JJ, *et al.* Definitive establishment of airway control is critical for optimal outcome in lower cervical spinal cord injury. *J Trauma* 2008; **65**: 1328–32.

24. Claxton AR, Wong DT, Chung F, *et al.* Predictors of hospital mortality and mechanical ventilation in patients with cervical spinal cord injury. *Can J Anasthes* 1998; **45**: 144–9.

25. Cotton BA, Pryor JP, Chinwalla I, *et al.* Respiratory complications and mortality risk associated with thoracic spine. *J Trauma* 2005; **59**: 1400–9.

26. Jackson AB, Groomes TE. Incidence of respiratory complications following spinal cord injury. *Arch Phys Med Rehabil* 1994; **75**(3): 270–5.

27. Fishburn MJ, Marino RJ, Ditunno J. Atelectasis and pneumonia in acute spinal cord injury. *Arch Phys Med Rehabil* 1990; **71**: 197–200.

28. Harrop JS. Tracheotomy in critically ill patients. *Mayo Clinic Proc* 80: 1632–8.

29. Romero J, Vari A, Gambarrutta C, Oliviero A. Tracheostomy timing in traumatic spinal cord injury. *Eur Spine J* 2009; **18**: 1452–7.

30. Goettler CE, Fugo JR, Bard MR, *et al.* Predicting the need for early tracheotomy: a multifactorial analysis of 992 intubated trauma patients. *J Trauma* 2006; **60**(5): 991–6.

31. Bouderka MA, Fakhir B, Bouaggad A, *et al.* Early tracheotomy versus prolonged endotracheal intubation in severe head injury. *J Trauma* 2004; **57**(2): 251–4.

32. Bishop MJ. The timing of tracheotomy. An evolving consensus. *Chest* 1989; **96**(4): 712–13.

33. Marsh HM, Gillespie DJ, Baumgartner AE. Timing of tracheotomy in the critically ill patient. *Chest* 1989; **96**: 190–3.

34. Shirawi N, Arabi Y. Bench-to-bedside review: early tracheotomy in critically ill trauma patients. *Crit Care* 2006; **10**: 201.

35. Kane TD, Rodriguez JL, Luchette FA. Early versus late tracheotomy in the trauma patient. *Respir Care Clin N Am* 1997; **3**: 1–20.

36. Moller MG, Slaikeu JD, Bonelli P, Davis AT, Hoogeboom JE, Bonnell BW. Early tracheotomy versus late tracheotomy in the surgical intensive care unit. *Am J Surg* 2005; **189**: 293–6.

37. Ahmed N, Kuo YH. Early versus late tracheotomy in patients with severe traumatic head injury. *Surg Infect (Larchmt)* 2007; **8**(3): 343–7.

38. Kollef MH, Ahrens TS, Shannon W. Clinical predictors and outcomes for patients requiring tracheotomy in the intensive care unit. *Crit Care Med* 1999; **27**(9): 1714–2036.

39. Frutos-Vivar F, Esteban A, Apezteguia C, *et al.* Outcome of mechanically ventilated patients who require a tracheotomy. *Crit Care Med* 2005; **33**(2): 290–8.

40. Arabi Y, Haddad S, Shirawi N, Al Shimemeri A. Early tracheotomy in intensive care trauma patients improves resource utilization: a cohort study and literature review. *Crit Care* 2004; **8**(5): R347–52.

41. Arabi YM, Alhashemi JA, Tamim HM, *et al.* The impact of time to tracheotomy on mechanical ventilation duration, length of stay, and mortality in intensive care unit patients. *J Crit Care* 2009; **24**(3): 435–40.

42. Griffiths J, Barber VS, Morgan L, Young JD. Systematic review and meta-analysis of studies of the timing of tracheotomy in adult patients undergoing artificial ventilation. *BMJ* 2005; **330**(7502): 1243.

43. Brook AD, Sherman G, Malen J, Kollef MH. Early versus late tracheotomy in patients who require prolonged mechanical ventilation. *Am J Crit Care* 2000; **9**(5): 352–9.

44. Chintamani KJ, Singh JP, Kulshreshtha P, *et al.* Early tracheotomy in closed head injuries: experience at a tertiary center in a developing country – a prospective study. *BMC Emerg Med* 2005; **5**: 8.

45. Sugerman HJ, Wolfe L, Pasquale MD, *et al.* Multicenter, randomized, prospective trial of early tracheotomy. *J Trauma* 1997; **43**(5): 741–7.

46. Gurkin SA, Parikshak M, Kralovich KA, *et al.* Indicators for tracheotomy in patients with traumatic brain injury. *Am Surg* 2002; **68**(4): 324–8.

47. Major KM, Hui T, Wilson MT, *et al.* Objective indications for early tracheotomy after blunt head trauma. *Am J Surg* 2003; **186**(6): 615–19.

48. Qureshi AI, Suarez JI, Parekh PD, Bhardwaj A. Prediction and timing of tracheotomy in patients with infratentorial lesions requiring mechanical ventilatory support. *Crit Care Med* 2000; **28**(5): 1383–7.

49. Lesnik I, Rappaport W, Fulginiti J, Witzke D. The role of early tracheostomy in blunt, multiple organ trauma. *Am Surg* 1992; **58**(6): 346–9.

50. Armstrong PA, McCarthy MC, Peoples JB. Reduced use of resources by early tracheotomy in ventilator-dependent patients with blunt trauma. *Surgery* 1998; **124**(4): 763–6; discussion 6–7.

51. Schauer JM, Engle LL, Maugher DT, *et al.* Does acuity matter? Optimal timing of tracheotomy stratified by injury severity. *J Trauma* 2009; **66**: 220–5.

52. Carrier FM, Turgeon AF, Nicole PC, *et al.* Effect of epidural analgesia in patients with traumatic rib fractures: a systematic review and meta-analysis of randomized controlled trials. *Can J Anaesth* 2009; **56**(3): 230–42.

53. Karmakar MK, Ho AM. Acute pain management of patients with multiple fractured ribs. *J Trauma* 2003; **54**(3): 615–25.

54. Saffle JR. Early tracheostomy does not improve outcome in burn patients. *J Burn Care Rehab* 2002; **6**; 431.

55. Holevar M, Dunham JCM, Clancy T. Practice management guidelines for the timing of tracheotomy. The EAST Practice Management Guidelines Work Group. *J Trauma* 2009; **67**(4): 870–4.

56. Holmgrem EP, Bagheri S, Bell B, Bobek S, Dierks EJ. *Utilization of Tracheotomy in Craniomaxillofacial Trauma at a Level-1 Trauma Center.* 2007 American Association of Oral and Maxillofacial Surgeons.

57. Lanza DC, Parnes SM, Koltai PJ, *et al.* Early complications of airway management in head injured patients. *Laryngoscope* 1990; **100**: 958.

58. Smoot EC III, Jernigan JR, Kinsley E, *et al.* A survey of operative airway management practices for midface fractures. *J Craniofacial Surg* 1997; **8**: 201.

59. Ng M, Saadat D, Sinha UK. Managing the emergency airway in Le Fort fractures. *J Craniomaxillofac Trauma* 1998; **4**: 38–43.

60. Bagheri SC, HAolmgren E, Kademani D, *et al.* Comparison of the severity of bilateral Le Fort injuries in isolated midface trauma. *J Oral Maxillofac Surg* 2005; **63**: 1123–9.

61. Thompson JN, Gibson B, Kohut RI. Airway obstruction in Le Fort fractures. *Laryngoscope* 1987; **97**: 275–9.

62. LoCicero J 3rd, McCaan B, Massad M, Joob AW. Retrospective study of all patients in an 18-month period in a CTICU. Prolonged ventilatory support after open-heart surgery. *Crit Care Med* 1992; **20**(7): 990–2.

63. Gaudino M, Losasso G, Anselmi A, *et al.* Is early tracheotomy a risk factor for mediastinitis after median sternotomy? *J Card Surg* 2009; **24**: 632–6.

64. Boyd AD, Bernhard WN, Sparaco RJ. Tracheal intubation and mechanical ventilation. In: Sabiston DC Jr, Spencer Frank C, eds. *Surgery of the Chest.* Philadelphia: WB Saunders Co., 1990; 256.

65. Marshall WG Jr, Meng RI, Ehrenhalt JL. Coronary artery bypass grafting in patients with a tracheostoma: use of a bilateral thoracotomy incision. *Ann Thorac Surg* 1988; **46**: 465–6.

66. Stamenkovic SA, Morgan IS, Pontefract DR, Campanella C. Is early tracheotomy

safe in cardiac patients with median sternotomy incisions? *Ann Thorac Surg* 2000; **69**: 1152–4.

67. Bacchetta MD, Girardi LN, Southard EJ, *et al*. Comparison of open versus bedside percutaneous dilatational tracheostomy in the cardiothoracic surgical patient: outcomes and financial analysis. *Ann Thorac Surg* 2005; **79**(6): 1879–85.

68. Westphal K, Byhahn C, Rinne T, *et al*. Tracheostomy in cardiosurgical patients: surgical tracheostomy versus Ciaglia and Fantoni methods. *Ann Thorac Surg* 1999; **68**(2): 486–92.

69. Petros S, Englemann L. Percutaneous dilatational tracheotomy in a medical ICU. *Intensive Care Med* 1997; **23**(6): 630–4.

70. Waldron J, Padgham ND, Hurley SE. Complications of emergency and elective tracheotomy: a retrospective study of 150 consecutive cases. *Ann R Coll Surg Engl* 1990; **72**(4): 218–20.

71. Heffner JE. The role of tracheotomy in weaning. *Chest* 2001; **120**: 477–81S.

72. Feinberg M, Ekberg O, Segall L, Tully J. Deglutition in elderly patients with dementia: findings of videofluorographic evaluation and impact on staging and management. *Radiology* 1992; **183**: 811–14.

73. Wakefield B, Holman J. Functional trajectories associated with hospitalization in older adults. *Western J Nurs Res* 2007; **29**(2): 161–77.

74. Donnelly F, Wiechula R. The lived experience of a tracheotomy tube change: a phenomenological study. *J Clin Nurs* 2006; **15**(9): 1115–22.

75. Craven D. Prevention and management of nosocomial pneumonia. *Emerg Med* 1992; **24**(16): 97–108.

76. Chastre J, Fagon JY. Ventilator-associated pneumonia. *Am J Respir Crit Care Med* 2005; **165**: 867–903.

77. Kollef MH. Ventilator associated pneumonia: a multivariate analysis. *JAMA* 1993; **270**(16): 1965–70.

78. Schneider GT, Christensen N, Doerr TD. Early tracheotomy in elderly patients results in less ventilator-associated pneumonia. *Otolaryngol Head Neck Surg* 2009; **140**(2): 250–5.

79. Baskin JZ, Panagopoulos G, Parks C, Rothstein S, Komisar A. Clinical outcomes for the elderly patient receiving a tracheotomy. *Head Neck* 2004; **26**: 71–5.

80. Graf JM, Montagnino BA, Hueckel R, McPherson ML. Pediatric tracheostomies: a recent experience from one academic center. *Pediatr Crit Care Med* 2009; **9**: 96–100.

81. Palmieri TL, Jackson W, Greenhalgh W. Benefits of early tracheotomy in severely burned children. *Crit Care* 2002; **30**: 922–4.

82. Principi T, Morrison GC, Matsui DM, *et al*. Elective tracheotomy in mechanically ventilated children in Canada. *Intensive Care Med* 2008; **34**: 1498–502.

83. Taira B, Fenton K, McCormack J, *et al*. *Timing of Tracheotomy in Pediatric Trauma Patients: A National Survey*. Abstract presented at Society for Critical Care Medicine 39th Critical Care Congress, Miami FL, January 2010.

84. Philippakis A, Hemenway D, Alexe DM, *et al*. A quantification of preventable unintentional childhood injury mortality in the United States. *Injury Prev* 2004; **10**: 79–82.

85. Fenton KE, Taira BR, McCormack, JE, *et al*. *Characteristics of Pediatric Trauma Patients Undergoing Tracheotomy*. Abstract presented at Society for Critical Care Medicine 37th Critical Care Congress, Nashville, TN: February 2009.

86. Taira BR, Meng H, Fenton, KE, *et al*. *Does Early Tracheotomy Lead To Better Outcomes in Pediatric Trauma Patients?* Abstract presented at The American Association for Surgery and Trauma 67th Annual Meeting, Maui, HI: September 2008.

87. Committee on Trauma ACoS. National Trauma Databank version 6.2. In: American College of Surgeons; 2008.

Intensive care unit tracheotomy care

Shaji Poovathoor, Eric Posner, James Vosswinkel, and Peggy A. Seidman

Case presentation

J. D. is a 38-year-old man who has spent the past 3 weeks in the surgical intensive care unit (ICU) after a motor vehicle accident. He underwent a tracheotomy in the operating room on day 7 of his ICU stay. He has been weaned from the ventilator and is now breathing humidified room air from a tracheotomy collar. He has a number 6 uncuffed tracheotomy tube in place and eats food by mouth. He is getting ready for discharge from the ICU and then eventually from the hospital. The patient would like the tracheotomy tube removed before he goes back to work.

Indications for tracheotomy

There are broadly three groups of patients with tracheotomy in an ICU setting: (a) those who required tracheotomy to bypass obstructive disorders (e.g., a foreign body that cannot be dislodged, infection, and tumors of the respiratory tract on vocal cords); (b) those being ventilated mechanically for a long period of time; [1–4] and (c) those who have undergone tracheotomy as a preliminary step in certain surgeries of the upper airway, chest, and head [5,6].

Approach

The two accepted methods for performing tracheotomies are open surgical technique and percutaneous dilational technique. The traditional method of performing a tracheotomy in a critically ill patient requires transportation from the ICU to the operating room, where the surgeon performs a surgical tracheotomy involving dissection of the pretracheal tissues and insertion of the tracheotomy tube into the trachea under direct vision. Percutaneous dilational tracheotomy has become more and more popular after the release of a commercially available kit in 1985 and involves the use of blunt dilatation to open the pretracheal tissue for passage of the tracheotomy tube.

Advocates of the percutaneous technique propose that the limited dissection results in less tissue damage and lowers the risk of bleeding and wound infection. Use of the percutaneous approach is often at the bedside in the ICU, which may lessen the associated risk of transporting a critically ill patient to the operating room. In a comprehensive meta-analysis Delaney *et al.* found that there was a reduction in wound infections with the percutaneous dilational technique compared with the surgical technique (OR = 0.28; 95% CI, 0.16 to 0.49, $P < 0.0005$) [8].

Tracheotomy Management: A Multidisciplinary Approach, ed. Peggy A. Seidman, David Goldenberg and Elizabeth H. Sinz. Published by Cambridge University Press. © Cambridge University Press 2011.

There was no significant difference in the incidence of considerable bleeding between the percutaneous dilational technique and the surgical technique. In addition, there was no significant difference in overall mortality between the two techniques.

The assumption is that complications may arise when a critically ill patient must be transported to and from the operating room. The data, however, is inconclusive and before a change in clinical practice is recommended, this would need confirmation in a larger, sufficiently powered multicenter randomized clinical trial. The general trend is to perform the "easier" tracheotomies at the bedside in the ICU where there are no delays associated with scheduling a surgical procedure [9]. Significant bleeding is rare, postprocedural infections are almost non-existent, and costs are drastically reduced. When compared with prolonged transtracheal intubation or surgical tracheotomy, the risks and complications are low.

The optimal time for performing a tracheotomy has not been clearly established. A common perception among critical care providers is that early tracheotomy may reduce the necessity for mechanical ventilation. One possible mechanism is that mobilization of the patient might allow improved pulmonary toilet and functional residual capacity, as well as avoidance of oversedation. Decreased airflow resistance and reduced dead space following tracheotomy may also contribute to accelerated weaning [9,10,13–16]. In a study of 20 patients, Davis *et al.* found decreased work of breathing per minute (8.9 ± 2.9 versus 6.6 ± 1.4 J/min, $P < 0.04$) and airway resistance (9.4 ± 4.1 versus 6.3 ± 4.5 cm H_2O/l per second, $P < 0.07$) after conversion of a translaryngeal tube to tracheotomy [17–21].

Early complications of tracheotomy

The overall complication rate is approximately 15% (range 6%–66%), and mortality is less than 1.5% (range 0%–5%) [25,26]. These complications could develop in the ICU after the procedure. The following is an overview of the early complications, which should be addressed in the ICU [20, 22–24, 27, 28].

Early complications

Hemorrhage

Sources of bleeding include small, superficial blood vessels at the tracheotomy site, granulation tissue, thyroid vessels, anterior jugular veins, and the innominate artery.

Operative hemorrhage is usually venous, originating from the anterior jugular venous system or the thyroid gland isthmus. Major hemorrhage can occur within several days or as long as 7 months after performance of a tracheotomy [29].

Management of minor bleeds

Incisional or stomal bleeding can usually be controlled by cauterization or packing around the stoma with petroleum jelly gauze. After examination and management of minor bleeding, the tracheotomy tube may be replaced.

In the ICU, careful suctioning following tube replacement should confirm resolution of superficial bleeding, or identification of secondary sources of bleeding.

If stomal bleeding or intratracheal sites do not account for bleeding, other sites should be considered. Gastrointestinal bleeding may be identified by placement of a nasogastric tube. The nasopharynx and oropharynx should also be examined for possible bleeding sources. Mucosal bleeding from radiation therapy may occur above the level of the tracheotomy stoma and be present in tracheal secretions.

Pneumothorax

Pneumothorax usually results from a breach of the pleural space as it comes up into the neck. If the pneumothorax is significant and causing hemodynamic compromise, then an intercostal chest tube must be placed in the ICU [30].

Tube misplacement and dislodgement

After a tracheotomy tube is placed, it is vulnerable to obstruction or displacement, which can be life-threatening [38]. Tube displacement may result from excessive patient motion, manipulation by staff on the patient, or inadequate tracheotomy tube securement.

Tracheal tube dislodgement can occur when traction is placed on the tube, especially when it is manipulated for ventilator connections. Long tracheotomy tubes can be dislodged inferiorly, causing the tip to abut the mucosal wall of the trachea, or obstruct at the level of the carina. Lateral neck X-rays may reveal that the tracheotomy tube opening sits against the tracheal wall or is obstructing the tracheal lumen. Manipulation of the tube or repositioning may resolve the obstruction. Tube displacement is especially dangerous in the first days after tracheotomy placement because the fistulous tract permitting tube reinsertion is not yet developed.

Obstruction

Any patient with a tracheotomy who develops dyspnea, difficulty in clearing secretions, or stridor must be suspected of having an obstruction until proven otherwise [14]. Plugging can occur from respiratory secretions and from blood or aspirated materials.

Management includes high-flow oxygen, and immediate tube exchange. Obstructions at the exterior tracheal tube opening can be manually removed. The tracheotomy tube should be suctioned to remove obstructing plugs. Use of a double-cannula tube may protect against obstruction caused by secretions. The inner cannula must be cleaned or replaced to prevent obstruction.

Tracheal cuff complications

Complications related to the tracheotomy tube cuff include cuff perforation, resulting in poor seal and increased aspiration risk; overinflation, causing pressure on or impingement of the tracheal lumen; and distention of the cuff distal to the tracheal tube, causing obstruction of the tracheal tube opening. Mucosal injury is much less common, as the use of low-pressure cuffs is standard. Pain with ventilation or swallowing, inadequate oxygenation despite correct tube placement, or presence of gastric secretions in the tracheotomy tube may indicate cuff problems. Appropriate measures include verification of appropriate inflation pressures (18–23 mmHg), and cuff position. If these symptoms persist, the tube should be replaced.

Other complications

Other complications include tracheoesophageal fistula, aspiration, and thyroid laceration. Less serious complications are subcutaneous emphysema, hypotension, and oxygen desaturation.

Care of tracheotomies in intensive care unit

Tracheotomy care can be divided into new vs mature tracheotomy care, but the ICU will most frequently be caring for new tracheotomy sites. Protocols for immediate post-tracheotomy care should include provide guidance for suctioning, patient comfort, ventilator management, and wound care.

Best practice advocates agree that a systematic approach to care ideally includes a "trach team" or at least an advanced care provider who is dedicated to these patients[31,32,33]. Many facilities do not have an adequate number of cases to merit dedicated personnel for these patients at all times. A reasonable approach is to have clearly assigned responsibilities and a method for documenting care in place.

Objectives for routine tracheotomy care:

(1) Prevent tube dislodgement
(2) Maintain skin integrity
(3) Maintain airway patency
(4) Provide patient comfort

Safety equipment availability

Emergency equipment that is appropriately sized for each patient should be near the bedside at all times. This includes extra suction catheters, a new replacement tracheotomy including inner cannula and tracheotomy stylet, endotracheal tubes, a stylet for the endotracheal tube, (b) and airway equipment that is routinely available such as a laryngoscope and blades, manual resuscitation bag, and capnography.

Tracheotomy patency

The inner cannula will need to be removed and cleaned due to secretion build up. The frequency with which this needs to be done will be patient and "age" of trach specific. Aseptic suctioning should be at done when assessment of the patient shows a need for suctioning. Given the risk for hypoxemia, tracheal mucosal damage, increased ICP among others, suctioning should be done only as often as needed given the clinical condition. Recommendations are often given for minimum time intervals, (i.e.at least once every 6 h) and more frequent suctioning is common in multiple clinical conditions, but there is no evidence-based guideline regarding absolute frequency of suctioning and it appears suctioning should be performed based on the clinical indications.

The suction catheter should be soft, not rigid, to decrease risk of mucosal damage, it should be smaller than 50% the diameter of the tracheal inner diameter to reduce risk of high negative suction pressures and potential hypoxia. Hyperoxygenation using the ventilator to control for TV and FiO2 is felt to improve oxygenation over manual valve bag ventilation. Closed suctioning systems may reduce the incidence of VAP (e). If a closed suctioning system is not in use, a clean sterile suction catheter should be used for all suctioning. Limiting each suctioning pass to less than 15 seconds and a maximum of 2 suctioning passes is recommended [31,35].

Cuff Pressure Assessment

Excessive cuff pressures have been associated with tracheal mucosal ischemia, cilliary tree dysfunction, tracheal erosion and stenosis. It is important to have the cuff inflated only if needed as for mechanical ventilation or aspiration risk[43]. Intracuff pressures can be measured using a spirometer attached to the air inlet port of the tracheotomy tube. Tracheotomy cuff pressures should be measured and documented to be maintained below 25mm Hg[32]. While not precisely equalt to the pressure being exerted on the mucosal wall, the cuff pressure is adequate for monitoring. Many patients are extremely sensitive to changes in cuff pressure and coughing is frequent when manipulating the cuff. Routine cuff deflation is not recommended.

All ventilator circuits should be supported so as to not pull on the tracheotomy site. This can put stress on the opening at the skin and internally on the tracheal wall and potentially dislodging the tracheotomy[31,36].

Patient Comfort

Although a tracheotomy is often more comfortable for the patient than an endotracheal tube, patients still may have discomfort that must be addressed. Post-procedure pain is lessened by the injection of local anesthetic, often mixed with epinephrine to reduce bleeding, at the incision site during the procedure. There is still incisional pain, however, that may require the use of systemic analgesics in the first few days after the procedure. Manipulation of the tracheotomy and suctioning are a frequent source of discomfort, and should be done with care as gently as possible. Sub-optimal ventilator settings and high cuff pressures often manifest as coughing or "bucking" and should be corrected. Finally, the abrupt discontinuation of sedatives and analgesics may precipitate acute withdrawal symptoms in the patient who has had continuous infusions of relatively short-acting medications that cause physiologic dependence.

Heating and Humidification

This is important to prevent drying of secretions, preserve mucocilliary function and prevent heat loss from dry inspired gases. Humidification systems should be mounted below the level of the patient to prevent aspiration of fluids in the circuit and changed weekly (unless soiled) to decrease VAP[34].

Site dressing and tracheotomy fixation device

Wound care is routine in many ICU's and will be touched on only briefly here. Tracheotomy sites are colonized with in 24 h and dressing changes are important for the health of the stoma. Maintaining a dressing under the fixation device but around the site is important for stoma hygiene but must be done with care to not dislodge the tracheotomy. Mature stoma's may need little to no dressing, but new tracheotomies should be dressed more frequently. There are many tracheotomy fixation devices commercially available as well as traditional "trach ties". There are no consistent evidence-based guidelines regarding changing of fixation devices due to the plethora of available devices. We suggest following manufacturer-specific recommendations and institutional protocols. Institutional guidelines and nursing protocols will guide practitioners as to frequency and type of dressing and trach ties used. At a minimum, an assessment of the site should be done every 24 h.

A tracheotomy can become dislodged in the ICU during routine care. Given the critical nature of a tracheotomy for patient viability, some guidelines are important for doing anything that involves moving the patient, particularly for an immature tracheotomy. These care events include but are not limited to:

- Moving the patient to change bedding or dressings
- Moving the patient for an X-ray, specifically a CXR
- Changing the tracheotomy dressing or fixation device

Utmost care must be taken that ancillary care providers in the ICU have all the assistance they need from the immediate care ICU providers to be sure that the tracheotomy isn't dislodged.

Weaning

There are many different strategies for tracheotomy weaning but there is no consensus on the optimal approach. A systematic multidisciplinary approach improves likelihood of success [39]. The aim is to develop goals for the individual patient, monitor ongoing progress and identify when further investigations might be required.

When the patient is being weaned from mechanical ventilation or from the tracheotomy tube itself, the use of a fenestrated tracheotomy tube and speaking valves or downsizing the tube may facilitate the decannulation procedure. The tube design allows the patient gradually to become used to handling secretions and breathing on his/her own. The tube can also provide the protection of a cuff if the patient should require supportive ventilation. When it is desired to have the patient breathe through his/her upper airway, the inner cannula is removed, the cuff deflated, and the outer cannula occluded by the decannulation cap. The capped outer tube with the cuff deflated will assist the patient to speak. One important factor to remember is to deflate the cuff, as total airway obstruction will occur if not done [26,46].

Conclusions

A patient with a new tracheotomy needs extra attention from all the ICU staff. Frequent assessment and suctioning, documentation of cuff pressures and site care are all necessary care plan activities. Complications may be more common in patients with tracheotomies than for those with an endotracheal tube. (g) Ongoing education is important to be sure the ICU staff understands the importance and reason for the workload and care necessary to maintain the tracheotomy. The delineation of a tracheotomy team to address these needs hospital wide is recommended but is frequently unavailable in small institutions(a). It is important for the nursing and respiratory therapy staff to have clearly delineated roles in the ICU for providing and documenting the care for these patients. Ongoing vigilance is essential for avoiding complications in patients with tracheotomies in the ICU.

The patient presented at the beginning of the chapter successfully underwent tracheotomy tube plugging, downsizing, and eventual decannulation before transferring to a rehabilitation facility. The stoma spontaneously closed over the following week.

References

1. Ross BJ, Barker DE, Russell WL, Burns RP. Prediction of long-term ventilatory support in trauma patients. *Am Surg* 1996; **62**: 19–25.

2. Lesnik I, Rappaport W, Fulginiti J, Witzke D. The role of early tracheostomy in blunt, multiple organ trauma. *Am Surg* 1992; **58**: 346–9.

3. Plummer AL, Gracey DR. Consensus conference on artificial airways in patients receiving mechanical ventilation. *Chest* 1989; **96**: 178–80.

4. Kluger Y, Paul DB, Lucke J, *et al*. Early tracheostomy in trauma patients. *Eur J Emerg Med* 1996; **3**: 95–101.

5. Baker SP, O'Neill B, Haddon W Jr, Long WB. The injury severity score: a method for describing patients with multiple injuries and evaluating emergency care. *J Trauma* 1974; **14**: 187–96.

6. D'Amelio LF, Hammond JS, Spain DA, Sutyak JP. Tracheostomy and percutaneous endoscopic gastrostomy in the management of the head-injured trauma patient. *Am Surg* 1994; **60**: 180–5.

7. Delaney A, Bagshaw SM, Nalos M. Percutaneous dilatational tracheostomy versus surgical tracheostomy in critically ill patients: a systematic review and meta-analysis. *Crit Care* 2006; **10**(2): R55.

8. Armstrong PA, McCarthy MC, Peoples JB. Reduced use of resources by early tracheostomy in ventilator-dependent patients with blunt trauma. *Surgery* 1998; **124**: 763–6.

9. Diehl JL, El Atrous S, Touchard D, Lemaire F, Brochard L. Changes in the work of breathing induced by tracheotomy in ventilator-dependent patients. *Am J Respir Crit Care Med* 1999; **159**(2): 383–8.

10. Rodriguez JL, Steinberg SM, Luchetti FA, *et al*. Early tracheostomy for primary airway management in the surgical critical care setting. *Surgery* 1990; **108**: 655–9.

11. Zeitouni AG, Kost KM. Tracheostomy: a retrospective review of 281 cases. *J Otolaryngol* 1994; **23**: 61–6.

12. Astrachan DI, Kirchner JC, Goodwin WJ, Jr. Prolonged intubation vs. tracheotomy: complications, practical and psychological considerations. *Laryngoscope* 1988; **98**: 1165–9.

13. Sugerman HJ, Wolfe L, Pasquale MD, *et al*. Multicenter, randomized, prospective trial of early tracheostomy. *J Trauma* 1997; **43**(5): 741–7.

14. El-Naggar M, Sadagopan S, Levine H, Kantor H, Collins VJ. Factors influencing choice between tracheostomy and prolonged translaryngeal intubation in acute respiratory failure: a prospective study. *Anesth Analg* 1976; **55**: 195–201.

15. Teoh WH, Goh KY, Chan CL. The role of early tracheostomy in critically ill neurosurgical patients. *Ann Acad Med Singapore* 2001; **30**: 234–8.

16. Davis K Jr, Campbell RS, Johannigman JA, Valente JF, Branson RD. Changes in respiratory mechanics after tracheostomy. *Arch Surg* 1999; **134**: 59–62.

17. Jaeger JM, Littlewood KA, Durbin CG Jr. The role of tracheostomy in weaning from mechanical ventilation. *Respir Care* 2002; **47**(4): 469–80.

18. Davis K Jr, Branson RD, Porembka D. A comparison of the imposed work of breathing with endotracheal and tracheostomy tubes in a lung model. *Respir Care* 1994; **39**(6): 611–16.

19. Lin MC, Huang CC, Yang CT, Tsai YH, Tsao TC. Pulmonary mechanics in patients with prolonged mechanical ventilation requiring tracheostomy. *Anaesth Intensive Care* 1999; **27**(6): 581–5.

20. Heffner JE. Tracheotostomy application and timing. *Clin Chest Med* 2003; **24**(3): 389–98.

21. Flint PW. Complications of tracheostomy. In: Eisele D, ed. *Complications in Head and Neck Surgery*. St. Louis: Mosby, 1993.

22. Waldron J, Padgham ND, Hurley SE. Complications of emergency and elective tracheostomy: a retrospective study of 150 consecutive cases. *Ann R Coll Surg Engl* 1990; **72**: 218–20.

23. Stauffer JL, Olson DE, Petty TL. Complications and consequences of endotracheal intubation and tracheotomy. A prospective study of 150 critically ill adult patients. *Am J Med* 1981; **70**: 65–76.

24. Pierson DJ. Weaning from mechanical ventilation: why all the confusion? *Respir Care* 1995; **40**(3): 228–32.

25. Brochard L, Rauss A, Benito S, *et al.* Comparison of three methods of gradual withdrawal from ventilatory support during weaning from mechanical ventilation. *Am J Respir Crit Care Med* 1994; **150**(4): 896–903.

26. Myers EN, Carrau RL. Early complications of tracheotomy. Incidence and management. *Clin Chest Med* 1991; **12**: 589–95.

27. Chew JY, Cantrell RW. Tracheostomy. Complications and their management. *Arch Otolaryngol* 1972; **96**: 538–45.

28. Jones JW, Reynolds M, Hewitt RL, Drapanas T. Tracheo-innominate artery erosion: successful surgical management of a devastating complication. *Ann Surg* 1977; **184**: 194–204.

29. Ameye F, Mattelin W, Ingels K, Bradwell R. Bilateral pneumothorax after emergency tracheotomy: two case reports and a review of the literature. *J Laryngol Otol* 1994; **108**: 69–70.

30. MacIntyre NR. Evidence-based ventilator weaning and discontinuation. *Respir Care* 2004; **49**(7): 830–6.

31. Ann McKillop RN MA "Evaluation of the implementation of a best practice information sheet: tracheal suctioning of adults with an artificial airway" **JBI Reports** 2004; **2**(9): 293–308.

32. Hettige R, Arora A, Ifeacho S, Narula A. Improving tracheostomy management through design, implementation and prospective audit of a care bundle: how we do it. *Clin Otolaryngol* 2008; **33**(5): 488–91.

33. Brilli, Spevetz *et al.* Critical Care delivery in the intensive care unit: defining clinical roles and best practice model. *CCM* 2001; **29**(10): 2007–13.

34. Dodek, Keenan, Cook, *et al*, Evidence-based guideline for the prevention of ventilator associated pneumonia. *Ann Intern Med* 2004; **141**: 305–13.

35. Mol DA, Du G, De Villiers T, Claassen AJ, Joubert G. Use and care of an endotracheal/tracheostomy tube cuff- are intensive care unit staff adequetly informed? *SAJS Intens Care* 2004; **42**(1): 14–16.

36. Littlewood. Evidence based management of tracheostomies in the hospitalized patient. *Resp Care* 2005; **50**(4): 516–18.

37. Kapadia, Bajan, Raje Airway accidents in intubated intensive care unit patients: an epidemiological study. Crit Care Med 2000; **28**(#3): 659–64.

38. Esteban A, Frutos F, Tobin MJ, *et al.* A comparison of four methods of weaning patients from mechanical ventilation. Spanish Lung Failure Collaborative Group. *N Engl J Med* 1995; **332**(6): 345–50.

39. MacIntyre NR, Cook DJ, Ely EW Jr, *et al*; Evidence-based guidelines for weaning and discontinuing ventilatory support: a collective task force facilitated by the American College of Chest Physicians; the American Association for Respiratory Care; and the American College of Critical Care Medicine. *Chest* 2001; **120**(6 Suppl): 375–95S.

38. Mohr AM, Rutherford EJ, Cairns BA, Boysen PG. The role of dead space ventilation in predicting outcome of successful weaning from mechanical ventilation. *J Trauma* 2001; **51**(8): 843–8.

39. Chadda K, Louis B, Benaïssa L, *et al.* Physiological effects of decannulation in tracheostomized patients. *Intensive Care Med* 2002; **28**(12): 1761–7.

Complications of tracheotomy

Steven L. Orebaugh

Case presentation

A 64-year-old patient with a history of laryngeal carcinoma and tracheotomy presented to the emergency department complaining of shortness of breath. Her other medical history included chronic obstructive pulmonary disease and hypertension. The patient related that she had been attempting to clean her tracheal tube *in situ*, due to the buildup of secretions within the lumen. She inserted a flexible cotton-tip applicator into the uncuffed tube and dropped it into the lumen. With her subsequent inhalation, only the proximal tip was visible. Afraid to remove the tracheal tube for fear the applicator would remain in the trachea, she left it in place and hurried to the emergency department. On arrival, her vital signs showed mild tachypnea, with a respiratory rate of 24, and oxygen saturation of 94% in room air, consistent with her previous levels.

Tracheal tube obstruction

Obstruction of a tracheal tube may occur from a variety of different causes. One of the most common is obstruction of the lumen by inspissated secretions [1]. The cough reflex or suctioning can help clear mucus, but a residual amount of this glycoprotein-rich liquid invariably leaves a coating on the tube's internal luminal surfaces. These secretions gradually lose their aqueous component through evaporation, and become dried, thick, and viscous. Unless the tube is periodically cleaned [2] (either by removal after scrubbing the internal lumen, or by frequent suctioning, ensuring a patent lumen) the buildup of such secretions may lead to a critical subtotal, or even complete, lumen obstruction [3]. Not uncommonly, tracheal erosion or irritation leads to minor degrees of bleeding in the airway, clots from which can contribute to tube obstruction. In addition, formation of granuloma tissue in the trachea because of mucosal irritation from the distal portion of the tracheal tube may result in symptoms of obstruction due to tracheal stenosis [4].

Tracheal tubes may become clogged in the postoperative period for a variety of reasons, including: tube misplacement or poor sizing (often resulting in the tip of the tube lying against the posterior tracheal wall and causing a "ball-valve" effect); thickening and inspissation of mucus in the lumen of the tube; and presence of blood or clots in the tube. This can be prevented with attentive nursing and hygiene, including frequent cleaning of the tube, use of humidified air or oxygen [2], use of tracheal tubes with an inner cannula that can be removed for frequent cleaning, and prompt measures to limit or stop bleeding, so that clots do not accumulate in the tube or airway (Figure 10.1).

Tracheotomy Management: A Multidisciplinary Approach, ed. Peggy A. Seidman,
David Goldenberg and Elizabeth H. Sinz. Published by Cambridge University Press.

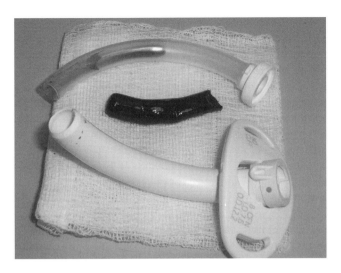

Figure 10.1 Tracheal tube and inner cannula after removal of large clot that completely obstructed the lumen.

This process will present with severe dyspnea, evidence of increased work of breathing, and high peak inspiratory pressures if the patient is receiving positive pressure ventilation. Breath sounds will become muffled or reduced in proportion to the decline in tidal volume that occurs. Patients breathing spontaneously will develop inspiratory and expiratory noise that coincides with airflow through the restricted lumen. An important diagnostic and therapeutic maneuver to help establish this diagnosis at the bedside is attempted passage of a suction catheter through the tube, in which instance the obstruction will limit or prevent its advance into the trachea. The diagnosis is largely clinical, and laboratory or radiographic data will not be particularly useful.

Therapy for this entity depends upon its severity. In milder forms, detected before critical luminal obstruction, irrigation with saline and suction with a catheter may serve to reduce the buildup and increase the patency of the lumen. Thus, attentive nursing care is essential. Removal of the inner cannula allows necessary cleaning, while maintaining ventilation. Alternatively, if the tract is well-established and there is no danger of losing the stoma for reinsertion, the tracheotomy tube may be removed, a substitute placed temporarily, and the offending tube soaked and scrubbed until the lumen is clean. In more acute settings, in which the process is well-advanced before detection, the patient may be in extremis, severely hypoxic, and/or hypercarbic before it is suspected. Attempts to assist ventilation with bag-valve apparatus will encounter extremely high resistance and pressures, as well as inadequate tidal volumes. If an inner cannula is present, its removal may help to re-establish ventilation. Rapidly attempting to pass a suction catheter through the obstructed tube will ascertain the diagnosis, but often will not ameliorate the severe obstruction, as passage of the catheter will not be possible. The tracheal tube must be rapidly removed under these circumstances, and replaced with a clean one (if maturation of the tracheotomy has occurred), or the patient may be ventilated and/or intubated from above in rapid fashion, to provide oxygenation and ventilation [1]. The last option will be impossible after certain surgical procedures, such as a total laryngectomy.

Foreign body in tracheal tube or airway

Because of its rigidity, and the acute angle of the lumen, foreign bodies introduced into a tracheal tube may lodge relatively easily. Some of these will have accidentally found their way into the tube, while others are put there intentionally, often in an attempt to clean the airway. Foreign bodies may be either firm or soft, each of which presents particular problems. Softer bodies, such as vegetable matter, may occlude the lumen in much the same way as mucus or clot, and present in the same fashion. However, attempts to push on or dislodge the body with a suction catheter or other instrument may result in its inward passage, producing a tracheal or bronchial foreign body. This may also occur if pieces of the tracheal tube itself are loose or broken, with distal migration resulting in airway foreign bodies [5]. In some cases, the body will break up and can be retrieved with irrigation and suctioning. In other cases, its retrieval will require more invasive management with rigid or flexible bronchoscopy [5].

Typically, patients are immediately cognizant that a foreign body is in the tracheal tube. When the body is firm in nature (e.g., cotton-tip applicator [or piece of one], or paper clip), it may not occlude the airway critically, unlike the softer variety. However, these can be very difficult to retrieve, and there is a risk with pushing any object into the tube, that the body will dislodge into the airway, creating a much more dangerous problem, probably necessitating bronchoscopy for removal. Thus, it is preferable to remove the tube, replacing it with another if necessary (or, managing the airway from above if the tracheotomy is immature), and gaining access to the foreign body outside of the patient. If the foreign body lodges in place but adequate ventilation is possible, the patient can be managed in the operating room, where the body can be extracted under controlled conditions.

Loss of airway with tracheal tube removal

One of the most feared complications in a patient with a tracheal tube is that the tube is inadvertently removed before the tract has sufficiently matured. This may occur from direct attempts by the patient to remove it, in the confused or demented patient, or simply during unrelated activities, particularly when a ventilator circuit is attached and the patient moves suddenly. The tract between the skin and trachea usually establishes in 5–6 days, and matures by about 10 days. Early removal or change of tracheal tube predisposes patients to this potentially disastrous complication [6]. When the tracheal stoma is well-developed and mature, replacement is usually not difficult, and little harm is likely to befall the patient in a short interval without the tube. However, when the tracheotomy has been recently placed, the tract will likely be immature and may not be easy to find when the tube has been removed. Even for those with experience, airway loss may occur when the tracheal tube is intentionally removed in the postoperative period. Tabaee *et al.* [7] found that, among chief otolaryngologist-head and neck residents surveyed regarding tracheal tube changes in the postoperative period, 42% had encountered airway loss during this procedure. If granulation tissue has formed in the airway, or tracheal stenosis occurred, airway loss might occur even well after the tracheal tube was initially placed [4]. Therefore, caution is always indicated during the initial change or removal of the tube.

Typically, patients present with dyspnea, tachypnea, and hypoxemia. If the tube is clearly out, the diagnosis is simple, but in some cases, the tube will appear to be in place beneath the skin but will actually be in a "false passage," not in the airway. It will be difficult to pass a suction catheter in this situation, and breath sounds will be reduced or non-existent. Sometimes, you may notice the patient breathing through the mouth and nose, if there is no obstruction of the upper airway. In such cases, loss of the tube may lead to life-threatening consequences, as replacement may be difficult and delayed [8]. When this occurs, it is important for the physician to concentrate on airway management from above. The ability to bag-mask the patient, or perform direct laryngoscopy with endotracheal tube placement, is essential. Some patients with tracheotomy will have undergone the procedure because of difficult laryngoscopy and/or intubation from above, and therefore will present a serious challenge. Others will have undergone the procedure because of failure to wean from mechanical ventilation, and intubation via the larynx should be less problematic.

Facial trauma, laryngeal removal at surgery, or a very large air leak through the stoma may all make face-mask ventilation ineffective or impossible in patients that have undergone tracheotomy. In such circumstances, ventilation through the stoma itself with a face-mask may be possible. A small pediatric mask should be chosen and placed over the stoma with an attempt to create a seal.

When replacement of the tracheal tube is attempted, surgical assistance is recommended, if available. In any case, appropriate tools for airway management and tracheotomy placement must be available, including tubes smaller than the one initially placed, and instruments on a tracheotomy tray, such as a dilator and tracheotomy hook, which can serve to open the tract for tube insertion. Placing the patient in a supine position, with a degree of neck extension will optimize both the opening of the tract and visualization, and, if present, pulling on the traction sutures may be all that is required to open the tracheotomy sufficiently to replace the tube. If visualization fails, gentle attempts to find the tract digitally may be successful. Generally, a tube one size smaller than the original should be placed [1]. When the tract cannot be visualized or opened, other options include placement of a bougie, or use of a fiberoptic scope to find the airway. When hypoxemia or deteriorating conditions do not permit such interventions, manage the airway with ventilation and tracheal intubation via the oral route.

Several factors might predispose a patient to loss of the tracheal tube. These include incorrect initial placement of the tube, a tube that fits poorly, loosening of the tapes that hold the plate of the tracheal tube, frequent coughing or vigorous motions by the patient, and a large neck.

When the tracheotomy patient undergoes translaryngeal intubation in these circumstances, attention to the level of tracheotomy is important. The orotracheal (or nasotracheal, if this route is chosen) tube must extend below the level of the tracheal incision, and the cuff adequately inflated to seal the trachea, or loss of gas through the stoma will occur, leading to inadequate ventilation.

Loss of the tracheal tube may have catastrophic consequences, but consistent use of traction sutures may prevent this, so that the tract can easily re-establish for replacement of the tube. Use of a correct size tube during initial placement is also important, especially if the patient has a short or obese neck. Suturing the base plate of the tube to the skin also reduces the chance of the tube coming out; therefore, also avoid tension on the tube from attached devices or during hygiene.

Postoperative hemorrhage

Hemorrhage may occur intraoperatively or immediately postoperatively related to lacerated vessels, or to oozing from a coagulopathic state. This will present as either obvious external blood loss, or as cough and increased suction requirements, yielding blood from the tracheal tube. In severe instances, tachycardia and hypotension may occur due to hypovolemia. Usually, the surgeon will be aware of this problem and will address it. However, if the hemorrhage becomes apparent hours later, the emergency or critical care physician may be the first to provide care. Minor hemorrhage that is evident externally can be treated with compression or packing. More severe bleeding, or bleeding that cannot be assessed and addressed externally, will require return to the operating room for cautery or ligation of vessels [9].

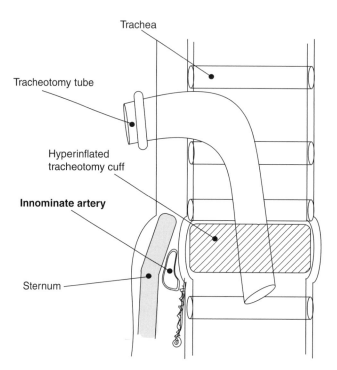

Trachea

Tracheotomy tube

Hyperinflated
tracheotomy cuff

Innominate artery

Sternum

Figure 10.2 Anatomy of the innominate artery and its relationship to the tracheal tube cuff. Erosion can lead to fistula formation with life-threatening hemorrhage. Overinflation of the tracheal cuff can tamponade the bleeding; passage of a longer tube with the cuff inflated below the fistula can prevent "drowning." Emergency surgical management is indicated.

Causes of later bleeding include granulation tissue, trauma from suction or changing the tracheal tube, progression of underlying neoplastic or inflammatory conditions, infection, and fistula formation. The overall incidence of postoperative hemorrhage after tracheotomy is approximately 3%, and about 10% of these cases are due to tracheo-brachiocephalic artery fistula [4] (Figure 10.2). In one study at a long-term care facility, the incidence of this life-threatening complication was 0.7% [10]. One-third of such cases present initially with a minor "herald bleed," which stops spontaneously. When the fistula forms fully, exceedingly brisk bleeding will occur, which will rapidly become life threatening [11,12]. Both the degree of hypovolemia and the blood welling into the airway (i.e., literally predisposing to "drowning") must be considered. Immediate overinflation of the tracheotomy cuff is recommended to provide a tamponade of the bleeding artery, allowing control until the patient can be taken emergently to the operating room. If this technique fails, insert a cuffed endotracheal tube, its tip placed below the site of hemorrhage to stop blood from entering the lungs. The tracheal tube must be removed, and digital pressure exerted on the bleeding vessel to control the hemorrhage [12], pressing the vessels against the sternum. Maintaining the patient in a position that allows drainage of the blood, and frequent suctioning are important aspects of treatment when hemorrhage occurs.

In both early and late hemorrhage, the severity of bleeding will dictate the interventions and the urgency of management. Any vigorous hemorrhage will require a return to the operating room for assessment and control, as well as protection of the lungs from aspiration of blood. The patient may require volume, blood products, or coagulation products as well, depending upon the cause of the bleeding and how quickly control can be established.

Subcutaneous emphysema

Subcutaneous emphysema is an unusual problem, which may result from excessive coughing, use of an uncuffed tracheal tube or an ill-fitting one with an air leak, or from tight closure of the wound with sutures, which will prevent escape of any air that comes around the tube [8]. This is particularly likely in a patient who has an underlying upper airway obstruction, as gases cannot vent from the larynx into the oral cavity. When percutaneous tracheotomy is performed, the risk of perforation of the posterior portion of the trachea is somewhat higher than with the open technique (see below). This may result in substantial air leak into the surrounding tissues. If subcutaneous air is localized and minor, correction of the underlying problem is sufficient, as air will reabsorb slowly without direct management. This may require replacing the uncuffed tube with one that has a cuff, replacing tight sutures in the wound to permit air egress, or addressing the patient's persistent coughing with an antitussive and effective suctioning [1]. Very severe subcutaneous emphysema can sometimes be addressed with placement of drains, or small incisions to permit air escape from large collections beneath the skin, but measures to address the underlying problem, preventing further air leak, are essential as well.

Percutaneous dilational tracheotomy

In recent years, percutaneous dilational tracheotomy (PDT) has been performed with increasing frequency in intensive care unit patients. This bedside approach reduces patient transport, bypasses logistic problems related to crowded operating room schedules, and is both technically easier to perform and cost-effective. This technique also appears to reduce long-term complications related to tracheotomy. However, acute complications may still occur, and the critical care physician or anesthesiologist taking care of intensive care unit patients must be aware of these [9]. Trottier et al. [13] evaluated PDT performance prospectively in a cohort of patients in a medical-surgical intensive care unit, and described a 12.5% incidence of posterior tracheal perforation with subsequent development of tension pneumothorax. This may be avoided by using simultaneous video bronchoscopy. Wise [14] reported the results of a survey sent to both trainees and established anesthesiologists in the United Kingdom. Acute complications described by this population included pneumothorax, hemorrhage, and loss of airway or misplacement of tracheal tube. A meta-analysis of studies comparing the open and percutaneous techniques described a lower frequency of postoperative bleeding and postoperative complications, as well as a comparable frequency of overall procedural complications with PDT [15,16]. Diaz-Reganon et al. [17] described an incidence of early postprocedural complications of 0.8% and late postprocedural complications of 1.1% with this procedure.

Other complications

Some other adverse occurrences in the wake of tracheotomy may occur, which are less likely to require urgent management, but are important nonetheless. Either long-term intubation or maintenance of an indwelling tracheal tube may result in mucosal irritation, inflammation, scarring, and tracheal stenosis [4,18]. Colonization of the tracheal wound is common, and frank infection may occur, although estimates of frequency vary widely [15,19–22]. Swallowing dysfunction is very common after tracheotomy, and may lead to malnutrition, or to aspiration of gastric contents with pneumonitis [23,24]. Poor fit of a tracheal tube with excessive pressure on the posterior tracheal wall may lead eventually to erosion or even a tracheoesophageal fistula [25].

Conclusions

(1) With acute tracheal tube obstruction, removal of the inner cannula permits cleansing and reopening the lumen while maintaining ongoing ventilation.

(2) Foreign bodies lodged in a tracheal tube may be removed at the bedside if accessible and ventilation is not impaired; otherwise, this should be addressed in the operating room.

(3) Management of a tracheal tube, which is inadvertently decannulated depends on the maturity of the underlying tract; if no tract is evident, attempts to reinsert should be abandoned in favor of translaryngeal intubation from above if possible.

(4) Most postoperative hemorrhage after tracheotomy is minor and may be managed with compression or packing at the bedside; severe hemorrhage (e.g., from a fistula) requires emergent attempts at tamponade and return to the operating room.

In the case presented at the start of the chapter, the tracheal tube was inspected and in the proximal end, a cotton-tip applicator was barely visible in the lumen. The lungs were remarkable for reduced breath sounds at both bases, and mild, scattered wheezes. Attempts to grasp the applicator through the tracheal tube with various types of forceps were unsuccessful, and some distal migration of the applicator became evident. The patient became increasingly uncomfortable, and she was transferred to the operating room for management. Subsequent attempts to remove the applicator under sedation were unsuccessful, and the decision was made to induce general anesthesia. After preoxygenation, induction of anesthesia proceeded with propofol and succinylcholine. The tracheal tube was removed, but the cotton-tip applicator remained in the trachea. This was grasped and removed with alligator forceps, after which a cuffed tracheal tube was placed. No trauma was evident within the visible tracheal lumen, and ventilation proceeded easily thereafter. The patient recovered uneventfully.

References

1. Walvekar RR, Myers EN. Technique and complications of tracheostomy in adults. In: Myers EN, Johnson JT, eds. *Tracheotomy: Airway Management, Communications, and Swallowing*, 2nd edn. San Diego: Plural Publishing, 2008; 35–67.

2. Lewarski JS. Long-term care of the patient with a tracheostomy. *Respir Care* 2005; **50**: 534–7.

3. Millar RC, Ketcham AS. Tracheotomy obstruction secondary to a T-adaptor. *Anesthesiology* 1973; **38**: 494–5.

4. Epstein SK. Late complications of tracheostomy. *Respir Care* 2005; **50**: 542–9.

5. Krempl GA, Otto RA. Fracture at fenestration of synthetic tracheostomy tube resulting in a tracheobronchial airway foreign body. *Southern Med J* 1999; **92**: 526–8.

6. Durbin CG Jr. Early complications of tracheostomy. *Respir Care* 2005; **50**: 511–15.

7. Tabaee A, Lando T, Rickert S, Sterwart MG, Kuhel WI. Practice patterns, safety, and rationale for tracheostomy changes: A survey of otolaryngology training programs. *Laryngoscope* 2007; **117**: 573–6.

8. Goldenburg K, Ari EG, Golz. Tracheostomy complications: a retrospective review of

1130 cases. *Otolaryngol Head Neck Surg* 2000; **123**: 495–500.

9. Grant CA, Dempsey G, Harrison J, Jones T. Tracheo-innominate artery fistula after percutaneous tracheostomy: three case reports and a clinical review. *Br J Anaesth* 2006; **96**: 127–31.

10. Scalise Paul, Prunk SR, Healy D, Votto J. The incidence of tracheoarterial fistula in patients with chronic tracheostomy tubes: a retrospective study of 544 patients in a long-term care facility. *Chest* 2005; **128**: 3906–9.

11. Rourke T, Tassone P, Clarke J. Emergency treatment of a hemorrhage from a tracheo-brachiocephalic fistula: a life-threatening complication of tracheostomy. *Eur J Emerg Med* 2008; **15**: 182–4.

12. Allan JS, Wright CD. Tracheoinnominate fistula: diagnosis and management. *Chest Surg Clin North Am* 2003; **13**: 331–41.

13. Trottier SJ, Hazard PB, Sakabu SA, Levine JH, Troop BR. Posterior tracheal wall perforation during percutaneous dilatational tracheostomy: an investigation into its mechanism and prevention. *Chest* 1999; **115**: 1383–9.

14. Wise H. Experience of complications of percutaneous dilatational tracheostomy. *Anaesthesia* 2002; **57**: 195–7.

15. Freeman BD, Isabella K, Lin N, Buchman TG. A meta-analysis of prospective trials comparing surgical tracheostomy in critically ill patients. *Chest* 2000; **118**: 1412–18.

16. Higgins KM, Puthakee X. Meta-analysis comparison of open versus percutaneous tracheostomy. *Laryngoscope* 2007; **117**: 447–54.

17. Diaz-Reganon G, Minambres E, Ruiz A, *et al.* Safety and complications of percutaneous tracheostomy in cohort of 800 mixed ICU patients. *Anaesthesia* 2008; **63**: 1198–203.

18. Sarper A, Aynten A, Eser I, Ozbudak O, Demircan A. Tracheal stenosis after tracheostomy or intubation: review with special regard to cause and management. *Tex Heart Inst J* 2005; **32**: 154–8.

19. Cole AG, Kerr JH. Paratracheal abscesses after tracheostomy. *Intensive Care Med* 1983; **9**: 345.

20. Henrich DE, Blythe WR, Weissler MC, Pillsbury HC. Tracheotomy and the intensive care unit patient. *Laryngoscope* 1997; **107**: 844–7.

21. Straetmans J, Schlondorff G, Herzhoff G, Windfuhr JP, Kremer B. Complications of midline-open tracheotomy in adults. *Laryngoscope* 2009; **119**: 1–9.

22. Stauffer JL, Olson DE, Petty TL. Complications and consequences of endotracheal intubation and tracheotomy: a prospective study of 150 critically ill adult patients. *Am J Med* 1981; **70**: 65–76.

23. Dettelbach MA, Gross RD, Mahimann J, Eibling DE. Effect of the Passy-Muir valve on aspiration in patients with tracheostomy. *Head Neck* 1995; **14**: 297–301.

24. Gross RD, Mahimann J, Grayhack JP. Physiologic effects of open and closed tracheostomy tubes on the pharyngeal swallow. *Ann Otol Rhinol Laryngol* 2003; **112**: 143–52.

25. Oliaro A, Rena O, Papalia P, *et al.* Surgical management of acquired non-malignant tracheo-esophageal fistulas. *J Cardiovasc Surg* 2001; **42**: 257–60.

Airway manipulation with tracheotomy

Daryn H. Moller, Slawomir Oleszak, and Ghassan J. Samara

Case presentation

An 85-year-old woman has a medical history significant for obesity, hypertension, coronary artery disease, chronic obstructive lung disease with recurrent exacerbations, and peripheral vascular disease. She was originally admitted to hospital with pneumonia, and after a prolonged intensive care unit stay and a failure to wean, she underwent tracheotomy and was transferred to a chronic care facility. After 3 weeks there, she returned to hospital with persistent fevers, increased white blood cell count, and an increasing oxygen requirement despite intravenous antibiotic therapy. A chest computed tomography scan revealed a multiloculated right-sided pleural effusion and significant consolidation of her right lower lobe.

The patient is scheduled for right-sided thoracoscopic drainage of empyema. The patient is awake and responds to commands. She is currently mechanically ventilated via a 6.0 cuffed tracheotomy tube. Her ventilator settings are pressure support 10 cm H_2O, positive end expiratory pressure (PEEP) of 5 cm H_2O, and 50% inspired oxygen. Physical exam reveals a Mallanpatti 3 airway with two finger breadths hyomental distance and limited neck extension secondary to multilevel cervical fusion. She has coarse breath sounds bilateral with decreased air entry noted at the right base.

- How do you provide for ventilation in an operating room setting? Does the lateral position affect your choice?
- How do you provide for selective lung ventilation for the surgical procedure? How are your techniques determined by the surgical procedure? By the patient condition?
- When do you intubate orotracheally versus use of existing tracheotomy?
- How do you manage intraoperative hypoxia?
- If removed would you recannulate the tracheotomy site?
- What are some potential complications of airway manipulation for this patient and how would they be managed?

Introduction

Within the past 30 years, there have been numerous improvements in advanced airway management. Much of this has been due to the development of new supraglottic ventilatory devices as

Tracheotomy Management: A Multidisciplinary Approach, ed. Peggy A. Seidman, David Goldenberg and Elizabeth H. Sinz. Published by Cambridge University Press.

well as new techniques in lung isolation. Growth of surgical technique has also expanded many of the traditional indications for lung isolation. However, many of the same concepts and indications remain and for patients with pre-existing tracheotomies, many of the newer devices and techniques can be applied. However, very little scientific research has been done in this area. The literature is populated by case reports of patients with specific or unique indications or conditions that required advanced airway management and how it was accomplished [1–3]. There are also several editorials about lung isolation methods and advantages and disadvantages to various techniques [4–6]. As a result, much of advanced airway management is based upon the clinician's comfort level and the various tools available to that person. Many of the techniques described in this chapter use currently available medical equipment that might be used in its intended application or in an off-label usage. The skill and decisions of the individual clinician remain paramount in providing safe airway control.

Airway manipulation basics

For patients with existing tracheotomy stomas or devices, there can be an almost limitless list of reasons for manipulations of the airway. For patients unable to tolerate decannulation because of respiratory failure or secretion management, routine tracheotomy changes are common and typically occur at a monthly interval. Various devices such as uncuffed or fenestrated tracheotomy tubes that are useful to patients in these chronic settings will provide a comfortable and functional airway that decreases dead space and allows for secretion management. If patients desire to vocalize, temporary occlusion of the tracheotomy stoma either manually or with a "speaking valve" will allow exhaled air to pass around the device or through fenestrations.

In these chronic settings, airway manipulation is often simply a matter of removal and reinsertion of the appropriate sized device. For patients that must be switched to full mechanical ventilation, a standard cuffed device can be exchanged for an uncuffed one directly. During reinsertion it is critical that the obturator be placed inside the device to assist in directing the tip towards the tracheal lumen.

An option for conversion to full mechanical ventilation would be removal of the tracheotomy device and standard oral–trachaeal intubation. In the setting of chronic ventilation in an intensive care unit, this probably represents the least comfortable option for the patient. However, for short-term usage such as the operating room environment, this represents a viable option. Oral–tracheal intubation may also be the ventilation method of choice for surgery involving positions other than supine, as it would limit potential pressure and torquing of the tracheotomy device. If this is not done, a flexible connector as shown in Figure 11.1 should allow for minimal pressure and motion of the tracheotomy device. For surgery involving the head and neck, such as ventriculoperitoneal shunt placement, orotracheal intubation can potentially remove the device or its securing hardware from the surgical field. Conversion to oral–tracheal intubation can be a simple matter of preoxygenation, removal of the tracheotomy device, and direct laryngoscopy and intubation. Intubation without an endotracheal tube stylet or one that was not severely curved anteriorly would be preferred, so the tube is not directed towards the existing stoma and potentially though it, creating a false passage. One could also intubate over a fiberoptic bronchoscope to assure that the endotracheal tube tip remains directed in the tracheal lumen. There is one case report of such tracheal injury related to orotracheal intubation in a patient with a fresh percutaneous tracheotomy [7]. Tracheal placement should be confirmed by the presence of exhaled carbon dioxide and bilateral lung auscultation.

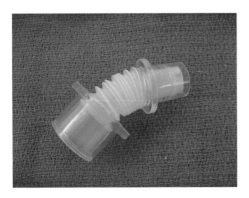

Figure 11.1 A flexible extension for use with tracheostomies. It has a male and female 15 mm tapered connector on either end.

For patients with total laryngectomies the simplest method of mechanical ventilation may be direct cannulation of the stoma with an endotracheal tube. An armored endotracheal tube has greater flexibility than a standard polyvinyl chloride tube and may be less traumatic to the stoma. It can then be secured to the neck with sutures or by cotton tapes or ties. A flexible adjustable tracheotomy tube (e.g., Bivonna tracheotomy tube) would allow direct cannulation of the site and has an integrated securing mechanism. An advantage of the Bivonna tracheotomy tube is that the cuff extends to the distal end of the tube. In the setting of a short stoma to carina distance, this minimizes the potential for endobronchial intubation.

It should be noted that a subset of the population will have rapid closure of the tracheotomy site upon decannulation due to collapse of soft tissue or granulation tissue around the Stoma. Granulation tissue might bleed profusely when manipulated, thus complicating airway control. Over relatively short periods (minutes to hours), contraction of circumferential scar tissue around even a mature tracheotomy site can occur making reinsertion of the original tube difficult or impossible. A Killian nasal speculum or dilator from a percutaneous tracheotomy kit is often helpful in re-establishing the stomal lumen. In these settings, changing tracheotomy devices would be preferred to oral–tracheal intubation.

Another short-term means to assist mechanical ventilation with an uncuffed endotracheal tube would be the use of a pressure support mode of ventilation. Assist control or synchronous intermittent mandatory ventilation will give a set tidal volume; gas leaking out around the uncuffed tracheotomy tube will frequently result in a low volume alarm, as the ventilator is unable to achieve its desired exhaled tidal volume. The use of pressure control with or without pressure support can increase tidal volumes and minute ventilation but the degree of assisted ventilation would be difficult to detect, as the exhaled tidal volume would not be reflective of minute ventilation. Monitoring of exhaled carbon dioxide or arterial blood gas analysis is useful in these situations but the clinician must be aware of a potential increased arterial to end-tidal gradient for carbon dioxide. If difficulty still exists in ventilation of the patient or neuromuscular blockade is needed, a short-term solution could be restricting the passage of gas through the larynx with packing. Care must be taken to place not too much packing as this may distort anatomy or compress vascular structures and do not leave any foreign material in the patient's oropharynx. In this setting, rolled gauze material made of a single continuous piece holds a significant advantage over individual gauze pads. Care should be taken to watch for gastric distention as positive pressure may force inhaled gas down the esophagus rather than out the oral–pharynx.

For recently placed tracheotomies (less than 2 weeks), any manipulation of the site can be fraught with difficulties. During a standard open tracheotomy, an incision is made in the tracheal wall to allow passage of the tube. Until wound healing has occurred and a fistulous track has developed, simple removal and reinsertion of a tracheotomy device has the potential to result in tube malposition. Many surgeons will place a stitch in the cartilaginous "flap" that is incised in the trachea and bring that inferiorly out to the skin. The theory is that traction on the suture will help to open the tracheal access site and direct a new tracheotomy and obturator into the tracheal lumen. This stitch is frequently removed after the first tracheotomy change at 2 weeks. For percutaneous tracheotomies, the opening within the wall of the trachea is merely dilated and no formal opening is made. These devices take significantly longer to develop a fistulous track and removal and direct replacement of a tracheotomy device is more likely to result in placement *outside* of the tracheal lumen. Ventilation of the false passage can result in significant subcutaneous emphysema or pneumomediastinum making subsequent airway manipulations significantly more difficult.

To minimize the potential for complications, tracheotomy removal and reinsertion can be accomplished with the aid of a guiding catheter. An adult and pediatric airway exchange catheter (3.7 mm and 6.5 mm respectively) can be inserted and serve as guides to replacement devices (Cook). Additionally, off-label use of devices have occurred, including pre-bent tracheal tube introducer catheters used for assistance in direct laryngoscopy and oral–tracheal intubation as well as a host of other devices ranging from airway suction catheters to nasogastric tubes. Care must be taken when threading a guiding catheter through a fenestrated tracheotomy tube, as it is possible for it to pass through the fenestration [8]. The guiding catheter could potentially injure the tracheal wall, as it is not directed parallel to the lumen. Pre-bending or shaping the catheter and careful attention to advancement in the face of resistance can minimize such complications. Regardless of the guiding device, confirmation of the tube within the lumen should occur, either by fiberoptic visualization or the presence of exhaled carbon dioxide.

Complications

Management of complications of tracheal site manipulations is directed primarily at restoration of a patent airway. If there is a question regarding the placement of any ventilatory device, confirmation should include measurement of exhaled carbon dioxide from the device. Fiberoptic bronchoscopy, although not as readily available, allows for direct visualization of the tube as well as the airway lumen. The presence of bilateral breath sounds is suggestive of correct placement, but in the spontaneously breathing patient may represent respiratory effort and air movement through the larynx, not via the surgical airway.

A technique to re-establish a lost surgical airway is assisted by a rigid long obturator. This is very similar to some emergent surgical airway devices such as Nu-trach by Portex (Figure 11.2). Here a long obturator is introduced through a skin incision and a ventilatory device directed over it. Confirmation of the obturator in the trachea is noted by ease of passage and tactile stimuli of the obturator against the cartilaginous rings of the trachea. In an emergent setting, a standard endotracheal tube stylet and downsized endotracheal tube can serve the same function. An airway exchange catheter can serve the same function as well as being able to provide a means of jet ventilation to maintain oxygenation [9].

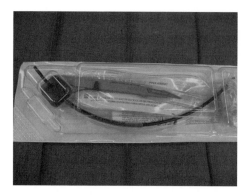

Figure 11.2 Airway device pictured can be used as an emergent cricothyroid device. (Portex® cricothyroidotomy Kit, Smiths Medical)

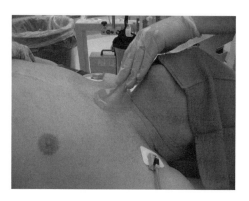

Figure 11.3 A laryngeal mask airway is placed over the tracheotomy stoma and an airtight seal formed with your hand. It allows for delivering positive pressure via a stoma without a formal airway device in place.

If the tracheotomy site has a well-developed fistulous tract, then assistance of ventilation can be accomplished via that site. Placement of a laryngeal mask airway (LMA) on the exterior surface of the neck and manual pressure around the inflatable cuff allows a seal to be formed and ventilation to occur (see Figure 11.3). Care should be used with this temporizing technique in a relatively fresh tracheotomy as positive pressure ventilation may result in subcutaneous emphysema and will make subsequent manipulations more difficult.

Lung isolation

Some of the indications for lung isolation are listed in Table 11.1. While traditionally thought of as indications for double lumen endotracheal tube placement, many of the requirements can be met via selective lung ventilation with a single lumen endotracheal tube and/or tracheotomy tube in combination with balloon occlusion of a major airway. One of the main differences between lung isolation techniques is the ability to provide selective ventilation versus selective isolation of ventilation. Another major consideration for lung isolation is concomitant disease of the upper and/or lower airways. An obstructing or even non-obstructing lesion in the airway can greatly affect an anesthesia provider's choice for lung isolation. Table 11.2 provides a generalized approach to lung isolation in patients. This by no means will cover every possible scenario that a clinician may encounter but provides global perspective of available options.

Table 11.1 Indications for lung isolation

Avoidance of cross-contamination between lungs
  Unilateral infection or hemorrhage
  Unilateral lung lavage

Control of ventilation
  Surgery on or disruption involving major airway
        Bronchopleural/cutaneous fistula
        Lung transplantation
  Selective lung ventilation due to unilateral lung disease or pathology
        Unilateral cyst/bulla in patient requiring mechanical ventilation
        Hypoxemia secondary to unilateral lung injury or edema
  Surgery in thoracic region requiring lung isolation for surgical exposure
        Open or video assisted thoracotomy
        Thoracic aortic surgery
        Robotic cardiac surgery
        Esophageal resections

Double lumen tube

Double lumen endotracheal tubes (DLT) have a long history of use in the anesthesia community. They have been the gold standard for elective lung isolation for years. A DLT can be quickly placed in most patients and its position can be confirmed with only clinical criteria. It allows not only for lung isolation during mechanical ventilation but also selective lung ventilation, suctioning, and lavage. However, for patients with pre-existing surgical airways, DLT placement is complicated by the presence of an existing airway (which must be removed) and the tracheal stoma.

During placement of a DLT, the bronchial lumen passes through the vocal cords with the curve directed anteriorly. As the tube is advanced, it is then rotated either clockwise or counter-clockwise depending upon whether it is a right or left endobronchial tube. During advancement down the trachea, the bronchial lumen can potentially become lodged in the stoma preventing advancement of the tube. Excessive force applied to a misdirected tube might cause injury to tracheal rings or surrounding structures. The chances of injury can be minimized by placing a fiberoptic bronchoscope through the bronchial lumen and advancing the scope down the trachea. The DLT can then be advanced over the fiberoptic scope that now serves as a guiding device. Though it is a possible mechanism of injury, it should be noted that no case reports were found in the literature of tracheal injury or false passage associated with this specific manipulation.

In general, one should not place a DLT through an existing tracheal stoma for the purpose of lung isolation. The distance between the skin entry site and the tracheal lumen is typically under 2 cm for an adult. A DLT is far too rigid to allow for bending at such a small radius. Doing so significantly increases the risk of injury to the posterior wall of the trachea as well as the anterior aspect of the upper tracheal rings. The external diameter of most tracheal stomas is also typically too narrow to permit entry of a DLT. However, there are case reports of this being done successfully [10,11].

For patients with total laryngectomies, the radius of curvature is far less and stoma diameter far greater. The limited flexibility of a DLT may place these patients at some additional risk for tracheal or bronchial injury, as the more probable site for injury is the posterior membranous portion towards which the DLT is being directed. In addition, it may

Table 11.2 Decision free for lung isolation techniques

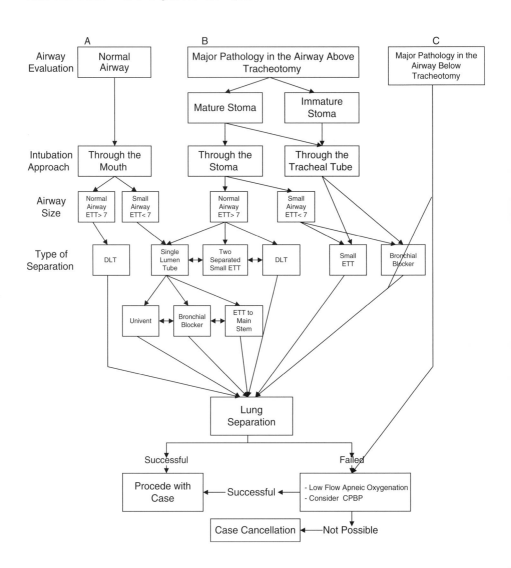

be difficult to secure a DLT, as the tracheal cuff may be located at the stoma site for some patients.

Endobronchial blockade

One of the primary modalities for selectively controlling lung ventilation is balloon occlusion of conducting airways. There are numerous commercial devices available such as the Univent endotracheal tube or Arndt bronchial blocker by Cook, designed specifically for this purpose. There is also a host of off-label uses of medical devices such as Fogarty embolectomy catheters. There is little scientific evidence to support the use of one device over another for a

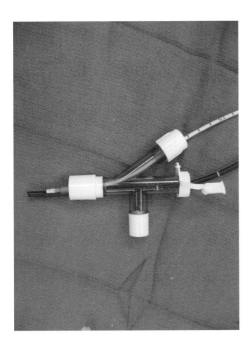

Figure 11.4 Pictured is a Cook bronchial blocker with the catheter "loaded" on a fiberoptic bronchoscope. The patient is connected to the left most port and the ventilator is connected to the lower port. To prevent leakage during positive pressure ventilation, the connector must be screwed tight around the bronchial blocker.

given situation. The selection is typically based upon the comfort and familiarity of the individual clinician as well as availability at a given institution. Some of the advantages and disadvantages of each will be discussed as well as clinical pearls for their use.

Effective endobronchial blockade is accomplished with the aid of a balloon inflatable catheter that can be passed through the ventilating lumen or alongside the airway device. When using the ventilating lumen of a tracheotomy, temporary removal of the inner cannula will generally increase the inner diameter by more than 1 mm allowing easier ventilation and passage of the fiberoptic scope. Care must be taken to reinsert the inner cannula at the end of the procedure, thus minimizing the chances of mucus plugging the tracheotomy device. The key pieces are the catheter itself and a connector to allow for ventilation and passage of the occlusion catheter. A Cook catheter is shown in Figure 11.4, which has a twist to seal connector for the occlusion catheter. Alternatively, a standard bronchoscopy connector can be used and both the catheter and bronchoscope passed through the same lumen. This is less desirable, as ventilation and catheter placement cannot occur simultaneously and withdrawing the scope through the same sealing diaphragm may result in malpositioning.

For patients with tracheotomies, an occlusion catheter can be introduced through the stoma alongside the tube or in an oral–pharyngeal fashion. This can be used in patients with a tracheotomy too small to accommodate the fiberoptic scope along with the balloon occluder. Oral–tracheal placement may be easier in the setting of a tight stoma or in a percutaneous tracheotomy and can be aided with simple direct laryngoscopy. Care must be taken during passage of the occlusion catheter so as not to injure the tracheal wall or damage the cuff of the tracheotomy tube, and deflating the cuff during passage should accomplish both.

Once the inflatable portion of the occlusion catheter is distal to the tracheotomy cuff, it must be directed into the appropriate mainstem bronchus. Owing to its more parallel alignment with the trachea, right mainstem occlusion is significantly easier than the left. For patients that have had their balloon occlusion catheter introduced via the tracheotomy,

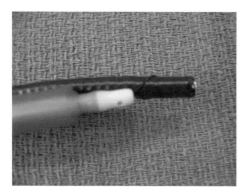

Figure 11.5 A bronchial blocker "loaded" on to a fiberoptic scope. The integrated monofilament snare is withdrawn slightly to fix the blocker firmly to the fiberoptic scope. When it is time to deploy the blocker, the snare is loosened and the blocker is advanced distally into the airway.

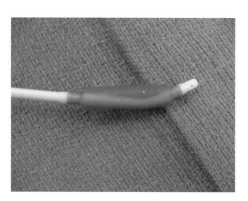

Figure 11.6 The tip of the bronchial blocker is gently bent without kinking or fracturing the plastic. Rotation of the device allows the user to "steer" it to either the right or left of the carina in similar fashion to a Univent blocking system.

the catheter can be guided with the aid of the enclosed monofilament loop. Typically, the fiberoptic scope is threaded through the distal loop and the whole assembly introduced into the trachea (see Figure 11.5).

The scope is then guided into the desired lumen and the occlusion catheter is then "threaded" over the scope and into the lumen. At this point, the scope is withdrawn partially to watch the balloon inflation to assure complete occlusion of the airway. In essence, this is exactly how the device would be used for patients intubated in standard oral–tracheal fashion.

In patients that require the occlusion catheter to be introduced alongside the ventilating lumen of the tracheotomy, a different technique is required. While it is theoretically possible to thread the fiberoptic bronchoscope through the guiding loop of the occlusion catheter to direct it, doing so within the confines of the tracheal lumen would be considered difficult at best. In these settings, a small bend (approximately 30°) can be introduced into the distal end of the bronchial blocker before placing it *in vivo* (Figure 11.6). Care must be taken not to fracture or kink the plastic of the catheter. With the distal 1–2 cm of the catheter angulated, rotation of the catheter from above can aid in directing it toward either mainstem bronchus. When watched from above, the catheter is advanced distally into the airway and the carina aids in direction down the desired bronchus. In either scenario, balloon inflation is watched from above to assure occlusion of the selected bronchus, but not of the trachea. Before surgical manipulation of the airway, care must be taken to withdraw the balloon occlusion

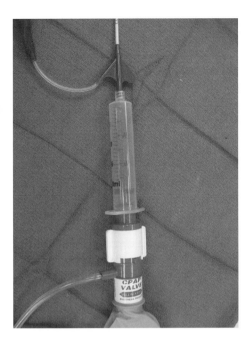

Figure 11.7 Continuous positive airway pressure can be supplied to the lung distal to the blocker by use of the included 15 mm tapered adapter to Luer Lock connector or via use of a 20 ml syringe. Either system can be hooked to the standard continuous positive airway pressure device commonly supplied with double lumen endotracheal tubes.

catheter as well as the internal guiding "snare." There is at least one case report of a snare being included in the staple line at a bronchial stump [12].

One of the main disadvantages of traditional endobronchial blockade is limited options to improve oxygenation during hypoxia. In traditional DLT ventilation, PEEP can be added to the ventilated lung and continuous positive airway pressure (CPAP) can be added to the non-ventilated lung, each in stepwise fashion. While PEEP can easily be added to the ventilated lung, there is limited ability to manipulate the lung distal to the occlusion catheter. If a Cook airway occlusion catheter is used, the central lumen (that houses the snare) may provide some ability to provide CPAP to the non-ventilated lung. By using the standard CPAP device supplied with most DLT tubes and a 20 ml syringe, you can convert the standard 15 mm tapered adapter connector to a Luer Lock connector to use on the distal central lumen of the occlusion catheter (Figure 11.7). The effectiveness of this setup may be limited by the length and relatively small diameter of the lumen and the potential for mucus occlusion.

Selective endobronchial intubation

In patients with pre-existing tracheotomy stomas, selective ventilation can also be achieved by direct placement of a single lumen endotracheal tube into the desired mainstem bronchus. Pre-bent oral and nasal endotracheal tubes are available in sizes as small as 3.5 mm internal diameter. As the typical oral to carina distance is 24–25 cm, these smaller diameter tubes should be placed via the tracheotomy stoma, as they do not have adequate length to reach the mainstem bronchi when placed orally. Using a fiberoptic bronchoscope with the endotracheal tube "loaded" on it, either bronchus can be selectively entered and the endotracheal tube advanced over it into the selected bronchus. Visualization of the placement should also be confirmed from *outside* the endotracheal tube to assure an adequate seal between the cuff and the mainstem lumen.

Selective lung ventilation is more of a technical challenge involving the right mainstem bronchus compared with the left mainstem. The right upper lobe bronchus has a variable attachment site to the tracheal–bronchial tree, which is anywhere from right mainstem bronchus to trachea proper. Because of this variability, it may be difficult to ventilate the right lung selectively without having the cuff of the endotracheal tube occlude the right upper lobe bronchus. In this setting, ventilation would be occurring in the right middle lower lobes only with a high probability for desaturation. Unfortunately, little can be done to solve this clinical dilemma.

Apneic oxygenation

In the setting of a thoracic surgical procedure, adequate operating conditions may also be achieved by brief periods of apneic oxygenation. Physiologically, as oxygen is consumed from the alveoli, its partial pressure drops. To maintain total atmospheric pressure within the alveolus, additional gas is drawn downward from the tracheal–bronchial tree. If the gas is pure oxygen, a patient may remain apneic for prolonged periods (15 min or more) without significant desaturation.

Case conclusion

Owing to the patient's history of cervical fusion and significant limited neck mobility, the decision was made not to attempt oral–tracheal intubation. The tracheotomy tube was removed and replaced with a comparable sized flexible endotracheal tube. A bronchial blocker was advanced down the right mainstem bronchus to allow for selective ventilation of the left lung. At the time of placement, it was noted that the patient had a high take-off of her right upper lobe. After placement of trocars for the video-assisted thoracic surgery, it was noted that the right upper lobe was continuously ventilated. Attempts were made in the surgical field to increase the insufflation pressures to 15 cm H_2O but the continued ventilation of the right upper lobe prevented adequate surgical exposure. Apneic oxygenation was attempted but the patient could only tolerate brief periods of less than 60 s. A decision was made to attempt selective blockade of the right upper lobe with an embolectomy catheter.

The tracheotomy cuff was briefly deflated to allow passage of a 7 French embolectomy catheter orotracheally alongside the tracheotomy tube. The catheter had been pre-bent at the tip and was advanced under fiberoptic visualization into the right upper lobe bronchus. The patient was disconnected from the ventilator temporarily to allow for collapse of the lobe and the balloon catheter was inflated in the orifice of the right upper lobe bronchus occluding it. The fiberoptic bronchoscope was carefully removed and the case proceeded. Intraoperative hypoxia was managed by the stepwise addition of PEEP to the ventilated lung. The final ventilator settings were inspired oxygen 100%, pressure control ventilation with $P_{inspired}$ 35, PEEP 12, with returned tidal volumes of 450 ml. At the end of the procedure, the balloons were deflated and catheters were removed intact from the airway. Based on the patient's high oxygen requirements, a decision was made to maintain mechanical ventilation postoperatively and the cuffed endotracheal tube was left in place.

References

1. Kraenzler EJ, Rice TW, Stein SL, Insler SR. Bilateral bronchial blockers for bilateral pulmonary resections in a patient with a previous laryngectomy. *J Cardiothorac Vasc Anesth* 1997; **11**: 201–2.

2. Vretzakis G, Theodorou E, Mikroulis D. Endobronchial blockade through a tracheostomy tube for lung isolation. *Anesth Analg* 2008; **107**: 1644–5.

3. Veit AM, Allen RB. Singlelung ventilation in a patient with a freshly placed percutaneous tracheostomy. *Anesth Analg* 1996; **82**: 1292–3.

4. Campos JH. Which device should be considered best for lung isolation: double lumen endotracheal tube versus bronchial blockers. *Curr Opin Anaesthesiol* 2007; **20**: 27–31.

5. Cohen E. Pro: the new bronchial blockers are preferable to double-lumen tubes for lung isolation. *J Cardiothorac Vasc Anesth* 2008; **22**: 920–4.

6. Slinger P. Con: The new bronchial blockers are not preferable to double-lumen tubes for lung isolation. *J Cardiothorac Vasc Anesth* 2008; **22**: 925–9.

7. Kazi ST, Ali MA, Donohoe BO. Accidental oro-endotracheostomy intubation. *Anaesthesia* 2006; **61**: 918–19.

8. Kasier EF, Seschachar AM, Popovich MJ. Tracheostomy tube placement: role of airway exchange catheter. *Anesthesiology* 2001; **94**: 718–19.

9. Mcguire G, El-Beheiry H, Brown D. Loss of the airway during tracheostomy: rescue oxygenation and re-establishment of airway. *Can J Anesth* 2001; **48**: 697–700.

10. Simpson PM. Tracheal intubation with a Robertshaw tube via a tracheostomy. *Br J Anesth* 1976; **48**: 373–5.

11. Seed RF, Wedley JR. Tracheal intubation with a Robertshaw tube via tracheostomy. *Br J Anesth* 1977; **44**: 639.

12. Soto RG, Oleszak SP. Resection of the Arndt Bronchial Blocker during stapler resection of the left lower lobe. *J Cardiothorac Vasc Anesth* 2006; **20**: 131–2.

Tracheotomy equipment

Dana Stauffer, John Stene, and Joanne Stene

Case presentation

You are working in the intensive care unit (ICU) and receive a telephone call from a colleague of yours working on the general ward. There is a patient with a tracheotomy tube having respiratory difficulty and they are requesting your assistance with the management of the airway. You quickly find your way to the patient's room and receive a brief report from your colleague. The patient is a 65-year-old man admitted yesterday for a major surgical procedure. He has a history of laryngeal carcinoma and has a metal Jackson tracheotomy tube in place. Upon assessment, he appears to be in moderate respiratory distress, breathing at a respiratory rate in the high 20s and using accessory muscles. The patient also had a history of congestive heart failure, and was observed overnight because of the large amount of fluid given the day before. He is now complaining of shortness of breath and you decide to move him to the ICU. You need to assist his respiratory effort; however, the respiratory therapist tells you this is not possible with a metal tracheotomy tube.

Functional components of a tracheotomy tube

Components of a typical disposable tracheotomy tube are illustrated in Figure 12.1. The **outer cannula** of the tube rests inside the trachea and houses the **inner cannula**. The inner cannula possesses a functional 15-mm adapter, which allows connection to a ventilator circuit or manual resuscitator. The inner cannula locks in place by twisting it in a clockwise motion. Tracheotomy tubes possess a curve that is approximately 90°, which allows the flange to fit evenly against the skin with the distal end of the outer cannula parallel to the trachea. The **obturator**, with its rounded tip, rests inside the outer cannula, in place of the inner cannula, and slightly protrudes from the distal end of the cannula. The function of the obturator is to protect against tracheal damage during insertion. Once the tracheotomy tube's outer cannula is inserted into the stoma, the obturator is removed and replaced with the inner cannula. It is common practice to keep the obturator at the bedside to facilitate reinsertion of the tracheotomy tube in case of dislodgement. The outer cannula maintains the stoma and patent airway while the inner cannula connects to the breathing circuit. The inner cannula can be easily removed for cleaning of secretions without losing the patent airway, which is maintained by the more permanent outer cannula.

An inflatable **cuff** near the distal end of the outer cannula seals the airway to improve positive pressure ventilation. Typical cuffs on modern tracheotomy tubes have a thin wall to

Tracheotomy Management: A Multidisciplinary Approach, ed. Peggy A. Seidman, David Goldenberg and Elizabeth H. Sinz. Published by Cambridge University Press.

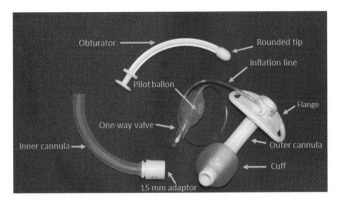

Figure 12.1 Components of a tracheotomy tube.

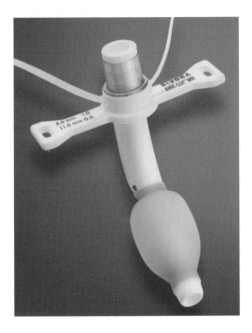

Figure 12.2 Bivona foam cuff tracheotomy tube. (Courtesy of Smiths Medical, Keene, New Hampshire, USA.)

facilitate the insertion and removal of the tube through the stoma and are designed to inflate to a high volume with low pressure. Foam cuffs (Figure 12.2) and low-volume, high-pressure cuff tracheotomy tubes are also available. Owing to longitudinal folds in the walls of high-volume, low-pressure cuffs, there is the potential that subglottic fluids will leak past the cuff into the lungs. Young *et al.* [1] found that low-volume, low-pressure tracheotomy tube cuffs reduced the risk of pulmonary aspiration in bench top models when compared with high-volume, low-pressure cuffs. Nonetheless, high-volume, low-pressure cuffs are found on most tracheotomy tubes.

In addition to enhancing positive pressure ventilation, a cuffed tracheotomy tube allows a certain degree of protection from aspiration and effective pulmonary hygiene. Cuffless tubes (Figure 12.3) cannot afford this protection, but may play a role in the long-term ventilation in patients with improved pulmonary compliance as identified by Bach and Alba [2]. This population of tracheotomy patients utilizing cuffless tubes can often phonate due to adequate oropharyngeal muscle strength despite insufficient respiratory drive to breathe without the tracheotomy.

The **cuff** is inflated by injecting air from a syringe through the one-way valve attached to a pilot balloon. The one-way valve is responsible for maintaining pressure within the tracheotomy tube cuff. It should be noted that integrity of a cuff should be verified before cannulation of the airway with the tracheotomy tube. Inserting air into the pilot balloon with a 10-ml syringe, placing in a bath of sterile water, and assessing for the absence of bubbles, is one method for ensuring the reliability of the cuff.

The **flange** of the tracheotomy tube stabilizes the outer cannula and prevents it from slipping through the stoma into the trachea. There are two pivot points between the flange and the outer cannula that allow for flexion of the outer cannula in the trachea. Tracheotomy tubes with adjustable flanges are also available (Figure 12.4). This allows for adjustment of

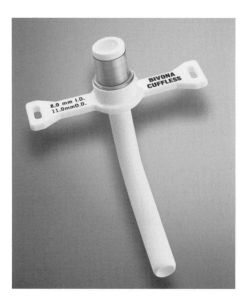

Figure 12.3 Cuffless tracheotomy tube. (Courtesy of Smiths Medical, Keene, New Hampshire, USA.)

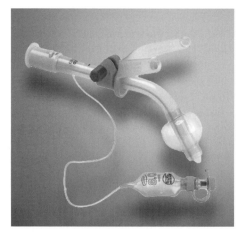

Figure 12.4 Portex tracheotomy tube with adjustable flange. Notice the thumb screw to tighten the flange to the outer cannula of the tube. (Courtesy of Smiths Medical, Keene, New Hampshire, USA).

the horizontal distance to facilitate proper placement of the cuff in the trachea in conditions such as obesity or glottic edema. Care must be taken to ensure that the outer cannula does not rotate within the adjustable flange causing occlusion of the tube by the tracheal wall [3]. Typically considered a temporary measure, adjustable flanged tracheotomy tubes should not be utilized for long-term use in patients where extra length is required. An extra-length tube with a fixed flange would be more appropriate for long-term use in these patients.

The tracheotomy tube is held in place within the stoma via twill tape or a commercially available soft tracheotomy collar looped through either side of the flange and passed behind the patient's neck. Clinicians must ensure the twill tape is loose enough so tissue necrosis or jugular venous compression does not occur. A good rule of thumb is one should be able to place two fingers between the securing device and the neck. The surgeon performing the tracheotomy operation frequently elects to secure the tube with four sutures passed through the slots in the flange. These sutures will need to be removed before the first tracheotomy tube change. Sutures should be supplemented with twill tape or tracheotomy tube fastener.

Special considerations and current controversies

Tracheotomy tube cuffs are designed to protect the lower airways from subglottic fluids and assist in maintaining a seal within the trachea to enhance positive pressure ventilation. However, even with high-volume, low-pressure cuffs, excessive pressures exerted upon the tracheal wall can lead to mucosal injury [4]. Monitoring inflation pressures within the tracheotomy tube cuff and not exceeding 30 cm H_2O can reduce the risk of tracheal wall damage. It is recommended that cuff pressures be monitored at least daily with the use of a hand-held pressure manometer [5]. In addition to commercially available pressure manometers (Figure 12.5), a syringe, pressure tubing, and stopcock can also be utilized to measure cuff pressures.

Underinflation of tracheotomy tube cuffs may lead to silent aspiration and should be avoided. An audible cuff leak is a sure sign that the tracheotomy tube is underinflated. Auscultation over the lateral neck may detect insidious, silent cuff leak. If a patient is connected to a mechanical ventilator, a low exhaled tidal volume (V_t) may be observed. It should be noted that pulmonary aspiration could lead to ventilator-associated pneumonia (VAP), which is the leading infectious complication in patients requiring mechanical ventilation [6]. Hence, it is important for clinicians to closely monitor cuff pressures on tracheal tubes.

High cuff pressures may be due to selecting too small a tracheotomy tube, resulting in the need to overinflate the cuff. Another reason for high cuff pressures is tracheal dilation. Utilizing a tracheotomy tube with a foam cuff is one method of decreasing the potential of damaging tracheal mucosa due to high cuff pressures. The foam-filled cuff, covered by a silicone sheath, is a large diameter, high residual design [7]. A syringe must be used to evacuate air from the foam cuff to facilitate insertion through the tracheal stoma. Once inserted, the pilot tube is opened to

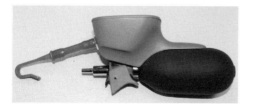

Figure 12.5 Commercial device for checking cuff pressures.

atmospheric pressure (there is no valve in the pilot tube of the foam cuff tube and the cuff is exposed directly to ambient pressure when the syringe is removed) and the foam passively expands sealing the trachea. Foam-filled cuffed tracheotomy tubes may be more difficult to insert due to the higher profile of the deflated cuff compared with standard tracheotomy tube cuffs. Proper sizing is important with the use of foam-cuffed tracheotomy tubes to ensure that neither leaks from too small a tube nor increased mucosal pressure from too large a tube occurs. Foam-cuffed tracheotomy tubes are often used in pediatric patients with tracheal injuries (e.g., tracheal malacia).

Materials

Modern tracheotomy tubes are typically designed for single use of finite duration and are constructed from medical grade biocompatible plastic such as thermosensitive polyvinyl chloride and silicone. As they are considered a disposable medical device, most manufacturers recommend tracheotomy tube usage not exceeding 29 days. The design and manufacturing of tracheotomy tubes are standardized according to the standards of the American Society for Testing and Materials (ASTM) [8]. The standardization documents reduce disparities between manufacturers who conform to the standards of the ASTM, greatly enhancing patient safety.

Disposable tracheotomy tubes allow for some flexibility within the trachea without causing tissue breakdown and necrosis. Tracheotomy tubes manufactured from polyvinyl chloride will soften insertion into the stoma due to a patient's body temperature. Metal tracheotomy tubes made from silver or stainless steel are less flexible, have been shown to corrode [9], and can cause irritation to tracheal tissue. Metal tracheotomy tubes (Figure 12.6) are also expensive to produce and cannot adequately protect the lower airway due to their cuffless design. Silver was used extensively in early tracheotomy tubes because of the wide availability of silversmiths who could fashion such tubes to various physicians' design specifications. However, the metal is soft, deformable, and tarnishes and corrodes in body tissues. Furthermore, some patients develop contact dermatitis to silver, which limits the use

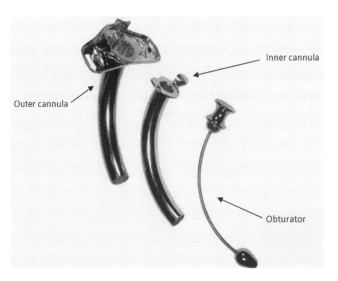

Figure 12.6 Metal tracheotomy tube. Notice the cuffless design.

Inner cannula

Outer cannula

Obturator

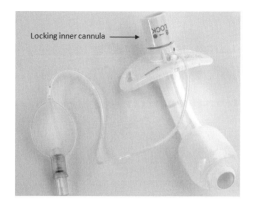

Figure 12.7 Dual-cannula tracheotomy tube. (Courtesy of Covidien, Boulder, Colorado, USA.)

Locking inner cannula

of this material in tracheotomy tubes. Stainless steel is somewhat more resistant to corrosion, but may contain nickel, which also causes contact dermatitis. Recently, silver tracheotomy buttons disguised as jewelry have been used to maintain patent stomas in patients with chronic tracheotomies [10].

Dual-cannula versus single-cannula tracheotomy tubes

Tracheotomy tubes are designed either with an inner cannula (dual-cannula tube) or without an inner cannula. Figure 12.7 demonstrates a dual-cannula tracheotomy tube. There are many advantages to utilizing a dual-cannula tracheotomy tube. Chiefly, the inner cannula can be removed if occluded with secretions that can impair the patient's ability to breathe. For long-term tracheotomy patients, the ability to remove the inner cannula for regular cleaning is important to facilitating good pulmonary hygiene. At one time, the daily changing of the inner cannula was considered essential practice; currently, this practice is not necessarily warranted in all patients [11].

Tracheotomy tubes without an inner cannula usually possess a standard 15-mm adapter (Figure 12.8). A single-cannula tracheotomy tube allows for a much smaller stoma size for a given internal diameter – the critical dimension for airway resistance – when compared with dual-cannula tubes. Table 12.1 displays the dimension comparisons for dual-cannula and single-cannula tracheotomy tubes. It should also be noted that the inner diameter increases when the inner cannula is removed from dual-cannula tracheotomy tubes.

Tracheotomy tube proportions

Tracheotomy tubes are designed to have standardized inside diameters, while the outside diameter will vary based on the manufacturer's proprietary classification system. The International Standards Organization (ISO) nomenclature determines the method for sizing all modern single and double lumen tracheotomy tubes. The French sizing system, used to measure the outside diameter of cylindrical medical instruments, is used to describe the outer diameter of the outer cannula of tracheotomy tubes. French sizing can be calculated as follows:

$$3 \times \text{Inside diameter (mm)} = \text{Maximum diameter (Fr)}$$

Table 12.1 Tube dimension comparisons for dual-cannula tube and single-cannula tube

	Dual-cannula		Single-cannula	
Size	Inner diameter (mm)	Outer diameter (mm)	Inner diameter (mm)	Outer diameter (mm)
6.0	6.4 (8.1 without IC)	10.8	6.0	8.3
8.0	7.6 (9.1 without IC)	12.2	8.0	10.9
10.0	8.9 (10.7 without IC)	13.8	10.0	13.3

IC=inner cannula.

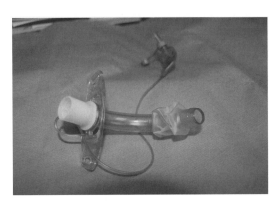

Figure 12.8 Single cannula tracheotomy tube with 15-mm adaptor.

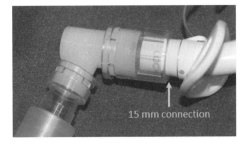

Figure 12.9 The 15 mm connection allows the interface between the tracheotomy tube and ventilator circuit.

It should be noted that aside from metal and specialty tracheotomy tubes, there is a stand-ardized 15-mm connector allowing a ventilator circuit or manual resuscitator to be attached to the tube (Figure 12.9). Customary tracheotomy tube proportions are listed in Table 12.2. Disposable tracheotomy tubes have the inside and outside diameter marked on the flange

Table 12.2 Approximate tracheotomy tube sizes

Jackson	French	Outside diameter (mm)	Approximate inside diameter (mm)
00	13	4.3	2.5
0	15	5.0	3.0
1	16.5	5.5	3.5
2	18	6.0	4.0
3	21	7.0	4.5–5.0
4	24	8.0	5.5
5	27	9.0	6.0–6.5
6	30	10.0	7.0
7	33	11.0	7.5–8.0
8	36	12.0	8.5
9	39	13.0	9.0–9.5
10	42	14.0	10.0
11	45	15.0	10.5–11.0
12	48	16.0	11.5

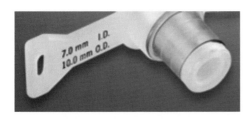

Figure 12.10 Inner and outer diameter marking on the flange of a disposable tracheotomy tube.

(Figure 12.10). If the tracheotomy tube is a double lumen, the published inside diameter is that of the inner cannula.

Tracheotomy tubes are produced in standard lengths and dimensions are ordinarily printed on the packaging. Extra-length tubes are commercially available and used in patients with tracheal anomalies. Extra distal length and extra proximal length tubes effectively bypass tracheal obstructions, a common cause of failure to wean from mechanical ventilation [12]. Figure 12.11 demonstrates an extra-long tracheotomy tube with dual cuffs, which allow alternating inflation and deflation of the cuffs to reduce the risk of tracheal trauma. While it is unknown how often extra-length tracheotomy tubes are used in patients, it has been suggested that both the stomal and intratracheal lengths should be made longer by approximately 1 cm [13]. Morbidly obese patients frequently require extra-length tracheotomy tubes.

The size selection of a tracheotomy tube is based on the patient's physical attributes such as neck size, anatomical variations, and age (Table 12.3). In pediatric patients, ultrasound may

Table 12.3 Tracheotomy tube sizes (pediatric to adult)

Jackson reference	Age
000–00	Premature
0	Birth to 6 months
1	6–18 months
1–2	18 months–4/5 years
2–3	4/5–10 years
3–5	10–14 years
5–9+	14 years to adult

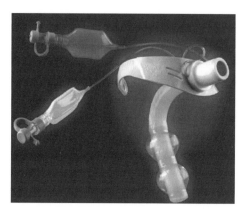

Figure 12.11 Double cuffed tracheotomy tube. (Courtesy of Smiths Medical, Keene, New Hampshire, USA.)

play a role in non-invasive determination of tracheotomy tube size [14]. High-resolution diagnostic ultrasound can be used to measure the tracheal diameter, depth of tracheal lumen from the skin, and angle of skin to trachea. These measurements are particularly useful in sizing tracheotomy tubes for children [14].

Typical sizes for women and men are 7.0 and 8.0 inside diameter respectively. This is associated with an approximate outside diameter and stoma size 10–11 mm. If the clinician selecting the tracheotomy tube selects a smaller outside diameter size relative to the size of the trachea, there is the risk of inadequately sealing the airway with the cuff. Selecting a tube with a large outside diameter may increase the difficulty in passing it through the stoma into the airway. Additionally, a large outside diameter will decrease the leak during cuff deflation making it difficult for the patient to phonate.

Tight to shaft tracheotomy tubes (Figure 12.12) possess a cuff that when deflated has the profile of an uncuffed tube. The tight to shaft tube offers the benefit of adding no distinguishable dimension to the outer cannula, increasing ease of use when inserting through the stoma. However, the main advantage of the tight to shaft tube is the reduced resistance when the cuff is deflated. This high-pressure, low-volume silicone cuff is designed for patients that require intermittent inflation for feeding interspersed by cuff deflation to allow use of the upper airway. The permeability of the cuff requires it to be filled with sterile water, as air will escape over time.

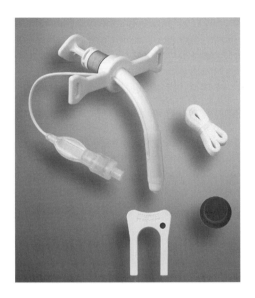

Figure 12.12 Tight to shaft tracheotomy tube. (Courtesy of Smiths Medical, Keene, New Hampshire, USA.)

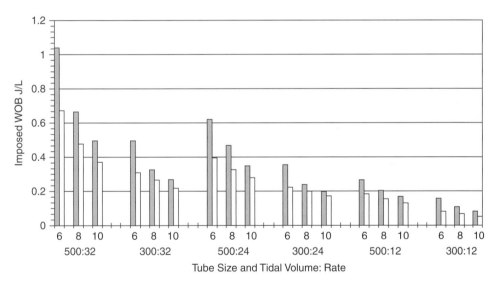

Figure 12.13 Imposed work of breathing (WOB) for Shiley size 6, 8, and 10 tracheotomy tubes, with tidal volumes of 500 and 300 mL and respiratory rates of 12, 24, and 32 breaths/min. Black bars denote WOB with the cannula in place. Open bars denote WOB with the cannula removed. (From reference [14], with permission from the American Association for Respiratory Care and RESPIRATORY CARE.)

The inside diameter of a tracheotomy tube is inversely related to the work of breathing imposed on a patient with an artificial airway. The smaller the tube sizes the higher the work of breathing, as demonstrated in Figure 12.13. Hence, when selecting a tracheotomy tube for a patient it is imperative to remember that a small tube in a large patient may lead to difficulty in weaning from mechanical ventilation. Tracheotomy tubes are often downsized when a patient is weaned from mechanical ventilation and breathing spontaneously. This downsizing of the tracheotomy tube requires the patient to have adequate muscle strength and the ability to generate enough negative inspiratory force to overcome extra resistance of the tube. In patients that are breathing spontaneously, who do not require connection to ventilator circuit, removal of the inner cannula may be beneficial as it increases the functional inside diameter of the tube, lowering the patient's work of breathing [15].

Fenestrated tracheotomy tubes

Fenestrated tracheotomy tubes are dual-cannula tubes with an opening above the cuff on the posterior wall of the outer cannula (Figure 12.14). Some tracheotomy tubes have a series of openings as demonstrated in Figure 12.15. When the inner cannula is removed, the fenestration provides a patent air passage from the distal intratracheal end of the tube to the vocal

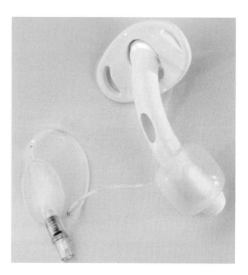

Figure 12.14 Fenestrated tracheotomy tube. (Courtesy of Covidien, Boulder, Colorado, USA.)

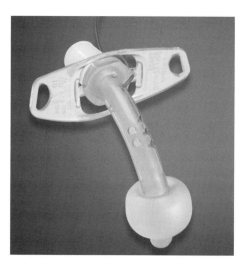

Figure 12.15 Fenestrated tracheotomy tube. Notice the multiple openings. (Courtesy of Smiths Medical, Keene, New Hampshire, USA.)

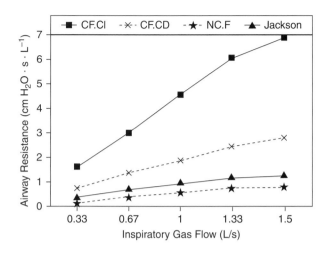

Figure 12.16 Graphic analysis of Raw during tracheotomy tube occlusion. CF, CI = cuffed fenestrated, cuff inflated; CF, CD = cuffed fenestrated, cuff deflated; NC, F = uncuffed fenestrated. (From reference [17], with permission from the American Association for Respiratory Care and RESPIRATORY CARE.)

cords and glottis. When plugging the proximal end of the outer cannula, the patient is forced to breathe through his glottic opening. Typically, a patient is suctioned, the inner cannula removed, cuff deflated, and proximal end of the tracheotomy tube occluded with a gloved finger to determine if the patient can inhale and exhale around the tube and through the fenestration. Once it is determined that a patient can breathe in this fashion, the tube is plugged with the cap supplied for this purpose allowing the patient to phonate.

One of the problems associated with fenestrated tracheotomy tubes is the misalignment of the fenestrations in the airway, leading to an increase in airway resistance. This risk may be minimized by utilizing a tube with multiple fenestrations [16]. Alternatively, the patient's anatomy can be aligned with the fenestration by measuring the distance from the skin to the tracheal lumen and selecting a tube with a fenestration corresponding to that dimension. An additional risk in using a fenestrated tube is the development of granulation tissue, obstructing the fenestrations and reducing gas flow [17]. Patients may also have an increase in airway resistance in cuffed tubes (Figure 12.16) regardless of tube inflation or deflation [18]. Hence, there is a movement towards using uncuffed tubes when capping tracheotomy tubes to decrease work of breathing during the decannulation process. Metal tracheotomy tubes can also be used for this purpose. Fenestrated tubes may be recommended in patients who have a high probability of requiring reintubation after decannulation. Furthermore, fenestrated tubes may be particularly useful in the patient undergoing tracheotomy collar trials along with use of a talking one-way valve, but needs full airway support with an inflated cuff on a periodic basis. During trial periods of cuff deflation, the fenestrated tube allows for a larger air passage around and through the tracheotomy tube decreasing the work of breathing.

Special purpose tracheotomy tubes and accessories

Low-profile tracheotomy tubes

These afford the active patient with sleep apnea or a laryngectomy a flange that is less noticeable. Low-profile tubes can be cuffed or uncuffed, with or without an inner cannula. Figure 12.17 demonstrates a low-profile tracheotomy tube that possesses a 15-mm adapter allowing for connection to a ventilator circuit. A silver locket has been designed to cover a permanent tracheotomy to disguise the metal tube [19].

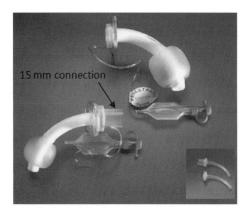

Figure 12.17 Low profile tracheotomy tube with 15-mm connection. (Courtesy of Smiths Medical, Keene, New Hampshire, USA.)

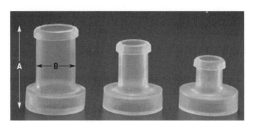

Figure 12.18 Tracheal stoma button designed to retain a tracheotomy valve. (Courtesy of Smiths Medical, Keene, New Hampshire, USA.)

Tracheal buttons

These provide stoma maintenance for patients who cannot be decannulated, by extending through the anterior neck to the tracheal wall. Figure 12.18 shows one commercially available button in various sizes designed to retain a tracheal stoma valve. Tracheal buttons are made from rigid Teflon or flexible silicone rubber and do not contain an inner cannula. Their primary function is to maintain the stoma and allow access to the airway for suctioning or emergency ventilation. Hall and Watt [20] found that patients with high spinal cord injuries benefited from tracheal stents due to reported significant improvement in relation to local discomfort, tracheobronchial secretions, and vocalization. The tracheal button has been used as an interim airway after tracheotomy tube removal. Long and West followed 163 patients with tracheotomy buttons placed after tube removal. Replacement of the tracheotomy button with a cuffed tube occurred 9.2% of the time, with 7.9% of patients discharged home with the button in place [21].

The Montgomery tracheal T-tube

This is another stoma maintenance device designed to support the tracheal wall (Figure 12.19). The design of the T-tube allows one limb to extend through the stoma, with the T portion resting inside the trachea, as demonstrated in Figure 12.20. A stopper is placed on the outside limb preventing the device from migrating through the stoma and into the airway. Importantly, in patients that require manual ventilation it is necessary to occlude the limb protruding through the stoma and use a bag-valve mask applied to the nose and mouth. It should also be noted that delivering inhaled anesthetic agents to patients with a T-tube might be problematic [22].

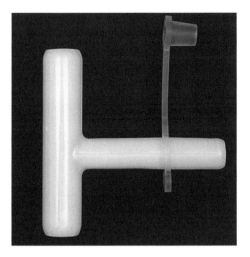

Figure 12.19 Montgomery tracheal T-tube (From reference [22], with permission.)

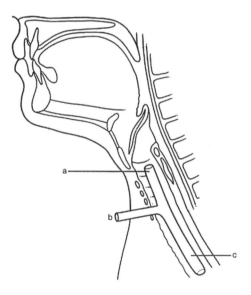

Figure 12.20 (A) Sagittal section of airway with Montgomery tube in place: ((a) short laryngeal part; (b) extratracheal part; (c) long tracheal part).

Tracheotomy tubes with subglottic suction ports

These have recently been introduced into the market (Figure 12.21) to combat the risk of VAP. The purpose of the port is to reduce the amount of subglottic bacterial-containing secretions, which may be aspirated into the lower airways leading to VAP [23]. One consideration in its use is that the suction port requires that tubes have a larger outer diameter.

Speaking tracheotomy tubes

These possess a separate pilot balloon that provides air to an outlet above the cuff (Figure 12.22). Compressed air directed through this outlet forces enough of an air stream through the vocal cords to allow phonation in a ventilated patient. This type of device requires the patient to coordinate to provide phonation. Furthermore, there is the potential for drying out of tracheal

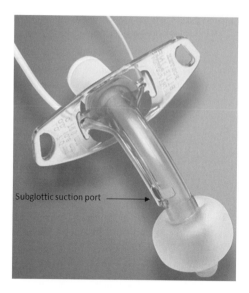

Subglottic suction port

Figure 12.21 Tracheotomy tube with subglottic suction port. (Courtesy of Smiths Medical, Keene, New Hampshire, USA.)

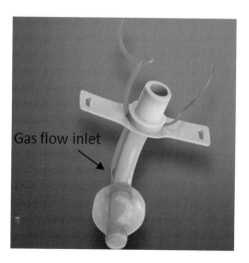

Gas flow inlet

Figure 12.22 Speaking tracheotomy tube. Arrow points to gas flow inlet that allows for phonation. (Courtesy of Smiths Medical, Keene, New Hampshire, USA.)

wall mucosa and secretions due to high compressed gas flows exiting the outlet above the cuff. The drying of secretions and occlusion of outlets has the potential to reduce the benefits provided by the speaking tracheotomy tube. Foam-cuffed speaking tracheotomy tubes are also available to clinicians (Figure 12.23).

Speaking valves

These provide an additional method of communication for patients with tracheotomy tubes. Figure 12.24 demonstrates one commercially available device. The speaking valve is placed on the external proximal opening of the tracheotomy tube. It can used on spontaneously breathing patients or individuals still requiring mechanical ventilation. Speaking valves are one-way valves that allow inhalation through the tracheotomy tube but block exhalation through the cannula forcing exhaled gas through the vocal cords allowing phonation

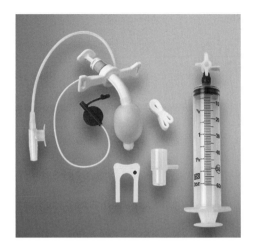

Figure 12.23 Foam cuff talking tracheotomy tube. (Courtesy of Smiths Medical, Keene, New Hampshire, USA.)

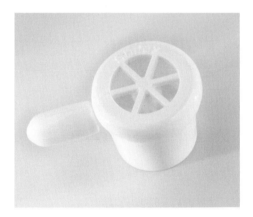

Figure 12.24 Shiley Phonate speaking valve. (Courtesy of Covidien, Boulder, Colorado, USA.)

(Figure 12.25). However, this process requires deflation of the cuff on the tracheotomy tube to allow airflow around it or use of a fenestrated tube without an inner cannula [24]. When utilizing a speaking valve in line with a ventilator circuit, measures will need to be taken to compensate for a decrease in delivered tidal volume due to the leak. In addition, positive end expiratory pressure may be difficult to achieve during this maneuver. Aside from improving patient communication, the deflation of the tracheotomy tube cuff and application of a one-way valve may improve swallowing physiology [25].

Percutaneous tracheotomy tubes

These are designed for insertion during the tracheotomy procedure that incorporates percutaneous dilatation. There are currently a number of products on the market, each with their unique characteristics. One such product is the UniPerc, part of a percutaneous dilational tracheotomy kit produced by Portex (Figure 12.26). The UniPerc is designed for patients with large necks with up to 50 mm of pretracheal depth. This particular tracheotomy tube has an adjustable flange to fulfill its objectives. Another design is the Cook percutaneous tracheotomy

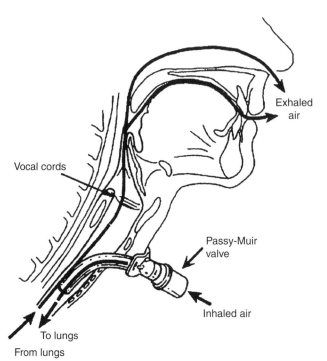

Figure 12.25 Passy–Muir valve mechanism of action. (From reference [24], with permission.)

Exhaled air

Vocal cords

Passy-Muir valve

Inhaled air

To lungs

From lungs

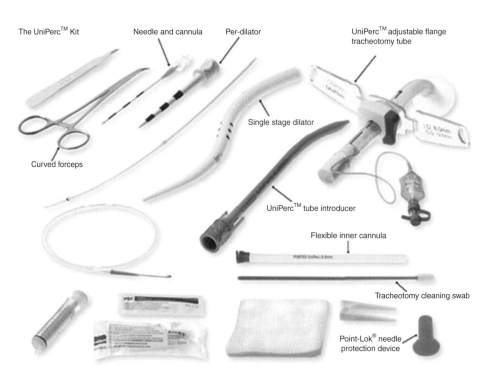

The UniPerc™ Kit

Needle and cannula

Per-dilator

UniPerc™ adjustable flange tracheotomy tube

Single stage dilator

Curved forceps

UniPerc™ tube introducer

Flexible inner cannula

Tracheotomy cleaning swab

Point-Lok® needle protection device

Figure 12.26 UniPerc, a percutaneous dilational tracheotomy kit produced by Portex. (Courtesy of Smiths Medical, Keene, New Hampshire, USA.)

introducer set used with the Shiley PERC tracheotomy tube, which has a tapered distal tip and inverted cuff shoulder for easier insertion [16].

Conclusions

The patient with respiratory distress that you transferred to the ICU is now doing better after being diuresed and receiving positive pressure ventilation. However, to ventilate him effectively you changed his metal tracheotomy tube to a cuffed, dual-cannula tube. You completed this tube change with the assistance of a colleague, and using the obturator, inserted the new tube without difficulty. Upon assessing breath sounds and establishing the patency of the inner cannula, you secured the tracheotomy tube with a velcro strap and checked the cuff pressure with a manometer. After receiving positive pressure ventilation for 16 h, you weaned your patient from the ventilator, and reinserted his metal tracheotomy tube before discharge.

References

1. Young PJ, Pakeerathan S, Blunt MC, Subramanya S. A low-volume, low-pressure tracheal tube cuff reduces pulmonary aspiration. *Crit Care Med* 2006; **34**(3): 632–9.

2. Bach JR, Alba AS. Tracheostomy ventilation: a study of efficacy with deflated cuffs and cuffless tubes. *Chest* 1990; **97**: 679–83.

3. Perkins GD, Freeman JW, Walia S. Cardiopulmonary collapse associated with malpositioning of an adjustable flange tracheostomy tube. *Resuscitation* 2006; **69**: 357–8.

4. Seebogin RD, van Hasselt GL. Endotracheal cuff pressure and tracheal mucosal blood flow: endoscopic study of effects of four large volume cuffs. *BMJ* 1984; **288**: 965–8.

5. Faris C, Koury E, Philpott J, *et al.* Estimation of tracheostomy tube cuff pressure by pilot balloon palpation. *J Laryngol Otol* 2007; **121**(9): 869–71.

6. Chastre J, Fagon JY. Ventilator-associated pneumonia. *Am J Respir Crit Care Med* 2002; **165**(7): 867–903.

7. King K, Mandava B, Kamen JM. Tracheal tube cuffs and tracheal dilatation. *Chest* 1975; **67**: 458–62.

8. American Society for Testing and Materials. ANS/ISO5366.1–00E Anaesthetic and Respiratory Equipment – TracheostomyTubes – Part 1: Tubes and Connectors for Use in Adults Approved as an American National Standard by ASTM International. 2003. http://www.astm.org/Standards/ANSISO53661.htm. (Accessed August 15, 2009).

9. Ayshford CA, Walsh RM, Proops DW. Corrosion of a silver Negus tracheostomy tube. *J Laryngol Otol* 1999; **113**: 68–9.

10. Tzifa KT, Jeynes PJ, Sheehab ZP, Proops DW. Cosmetic tracheostomy locket: an attempt to improve the aesthetic component of tracheostomy tubes. *J Laryngol Otol* 2000; **114**: 777–8.

11. Burns SM, Spilman S, Wilmoth D, *et al.* Are frequent inner cannula changes necessary? A pilot study. *Heart Lung* 1998; **27**: 58–62.

12. Rumbak MJ, Walsh FW, Anderson WM, *et al.* Significant tracheal obstruction causing failure to wean in patients requiring prolonged mechanical ventilation: a forgotten complication of long-term mechanical ventilation. *Chest* 1999; **115**(4): 1092–5.

13. Mallick A, Bondenham A, Elliot S, Oram J. An investigation into the length of standard tracheostomy tubes in critical care patients. *Anaesthesia* 2008; **63**: 302–6.

14. Hardee PSGF, Ng SY, Cashman M. Ultrasound imagining in the preoperative estimation of the size of a tracheostomy tube required in specialized operation in children. *Br J Oral Maxillofac Surg* 2003; **41**: 312–16.

15. Cowan T, Op'tHolt TB, Gegenheimer C, et al. Effect of inner cannula removal on the work of breathing imposed by tracheostomy tubes: a bench study. *Respir Care* 2001; **46**(5): 460–5.

16. Hess DR. Tracheostomy tubes and related appliances. *Respir Care* 2005; **50**(4): 497–510.

17. Siddharth P, Mazzarella L. Granuloma associated with fenestrated tracheostomy tubes. *Am J Surg* 1985; **150**(2): 279–80.

18. Beard B, Monaco MJ. Tracheostomy discontinuation: impact of tube selection on resistance during tube occlusion. *Respir Care* 1993; **38**(3): 267–70.

19. Burton GG, Hodgin JE, Ward JJ. *Respiratory Care: A Guide to Clinical Practice*. Philadelphia: Lippincott-Raven Publishers, 1997: 582.

20. Hall AM, Watt JWH. The use of tracheal stoma stents in high spinal cord injury: a patient friendly alternative to long-term tracheostomy tubes. *Spinal Cord* 2008; **46** (11): 753–5.

21. Long J, West G. The Olympic trach-button as an interim airway following tracheostomy tube removal. *Respir Care* 1981; **26**: 1269–72.

22. Guha A, Mostafa SM, Kendall JB. The Montgomery T-tube: anaesthetic problems and solutions. *Br J Anaesth* 2001; **87**(5): 787–90.

23. Valles J, Artigas A, Rello J, et al. Continuous aspiration of subglottic secretions in preventing ventilator-associated pneumonia. *Ann Intern Med* 1995; **122**(3): 179–86.

24. Hodder RV. A 55-year-old patient with advanced COPD, tracheostomy tube, and sudden respiratory distress. *Chest* 2002; **121**: 279–80.

25. Suiter DM, McCullough GH, Powell PW. Effects of cuff deflation and one-way tracheostomy speaking valve placement on swallow physiology. *Dysphagia* 2003; **18**: 285–92.

Chapter 13

Care of the patient with a tracheotomy

Margaret Wojnar and Jonathan D. McGinn

Case presentation

P.F. is a 25-year-old man with a history of congenital central hypoventilation syndrome and a left hypoplastic lung, which was later resected secondary to recurrent infections. He has undergone chronic nocturnal ventilation since he was 6 months of age. During the day, he caps his tracheotomy and keeps his cuff deflated. At night, he uses volume ventilation and a heat and moisture exchange (HME) humidification system. Recently, he was admitted to hospital for pneumonia. His oxygen requirement was increased but he was comfortable off the ventilator during the day so his home routine was continued.

- Should his home routine be maintained?
- What problems might be encountered?
- What are the options of care?
- Are there evidence-based data to support the therapeutic decisions?

To answer the questions regarding this patient's care, one has to understand issues normally encountered with a chronic tracheotomy. The initial and continued reason for the tracheotomy will determine some of the monitoring issues. The need for continuous ventilation does not necessarily change the problem list, but rather it may expand it. Key issues for the chronic tracheotomy patient include secretions and their control, humidification, tracheotomy site care, and proper tracheotomy tube fitting. The patient will encounter different needs from home to hospital and these will vary depending on the reason for the tracheotomy. Speaking and swallowing with a tracheotomy are covered in another section.

Introduction

The tracheotomized patient faces many challenges in maintaining a semblance of normal airway function. When ventilation (either assisted or spontaneous) is performed via the tracheotomy, several normal airway functions must be augmented or replaced. In a typical nasotracheal respiring patient, the inspired air is humidified and warmed to appropriate physiologic parameters by the nasal mucosa. This includes 100% humidity and body temperature. Without passage of the air through the nose, these functions are missing. The consequences to the lower airways can include thickening of tracheobronchial secretions, mucus plugging, tracheitis sicca, and bleeding.

Tracheotomy Management: A Multidisciplinary Approach, ed. Peggy A. Seidman, David Goldenberg and Elizabeth H. Sinz. Published by Cambridge University Press.
© Cambridge University Press 2011.

Secretions

Normal airway secretion management and reduction of excessive or tenacious secretions are important in the care of a patient with a chronic tracheotomy. Secretions are substances normally produced and released by cells, and in the respiratory tract are primarily represented by mucus. When this mucus is expectorated, it is called sputum. Mucus is key part of the defense mechanism for normal airways. When we breathe, millions of airborne particles are inhaled along with the inspired air. Mucus, a viscoelastic gel, forms a thin film on the surface of the airways to hydrate the epithelium but also entraps viruses, bacteria, and other foreign matter [1]. The respiratory epithelium of the lung is ciliated from the glottis to the level of the respiratory bronchioles. These cilia provide a propulsive action to the mucus blanket in a process intended to transport this foreign material from the airway before these damaging substances injure the lung.

Composition of mucus

Airway mucus is complex and made up of a number of beneficial substances forming a bi-layer above the cilia. The lower layer is more aqueous, sometimes referred to as the sol phase, and is in direct contact with the cilia. The upper layer is the gel layer that floats on the aqueous layer. A thin layer of surfactant lies between the sol and gel phase with the surfactant facilitating mucus spread. This organized structure to the mucociliary blanket is believed to be important for it to function. Mucus also detoxifies many noxious molecules with anti-oxidant, antiprotease, and antimicrobial properties. Mucin glycoprotein, the major macro-molecule of mucus, can be subdivided into three major families: secreted gel-forming mucins; membrane-associated mucins; and non-gel-forming mucins [2]. There is a vast literature base on the chemical and biophysical properties of mucus. Mucus production, storage, and release have been characterized. There are at least 20 human genes identified for mucus called MUC genes [2], nine of which are expressed in the respiratory tract. Mucins are upregulated by viruses, bacteria, various inflammatory mediators, irritants, and toxins. Specific mediators upregulate specific genes, such as tumor necrosis factor for MUC5AC, which is an active area of investigation [2].

The interaction of mucus with cilia and airflow allows us to understand the behavior of airway secretions. Understanding the observed properties of elasticity, viscosity, and shearing of mucus are key to determining what interventions might work more effectively. The secretions can be thick or thin, scarce or copious. In certain pathologic states such as asthma, chronic obstruction pulmonary disease, and cystic fibrosis (CF) [1–4], the properties of the mucus changes as the components of the secretions change. Mucus that is elastic and not as viscous is better suited for clearance by ciliary transport, but not as well by coughing. Mucus that has a dominant thick layer, and is more viscous than elastic, is more suited for removal by coughing. Knowing the properties of mucus before initiating therapy might then be helpful. What is known in the laboratory has not completely translated to the bedside, though some progress has been made. An example is in CF, where sputum contains little mucin but has other macromolecules that include DNA, lipids, proteoglycans, and filamentous actin [2]. DNA is released by necrotic neutrophils and increases mucus viscosity. Dornase alfa, a recombinant human deoxyribonuclease, is used to break up CF mucus theoretically by degrading DNA and actin found in the sputum of patients with CF.

Secretion removal

Therapies available to augment secretion removal can be divided into four different groups: expectorants; mucolytics; mucokinetic agents; and mucoregulators [3]. The expectorant class hydrates and increases the volume of the secretions. They may also act as an irritant and induce coughing to remove mucus. The mucolytic class reduces the viscosity of the secretions mainly by dissociating disulfide bonds or by breaking bonds in DNA and actin. The mucokinetic agents work by increasing ciliary beat efficiency or by changing adherence of mucus to the epithelium. The mucoregulator class interrupts production and reduces the secretion of mucus. Controversy arises on the true action of a number of agents used for mucus removal. There are currently compounds in development where the mechanism of action is either unknown, incompletely understood, or incompletely defined [3]. Many medications have more than one effect. N-acetylcysteine, for example, is thought to have mucolytic properties as well as antioxidant activities. However, data from clinical trials are ambiguous. Oral N-acetylcysteine results varied from no effect on dyspnea, cough, mucus production, or lung function to reduced thickness of sputum and severity of cough as well as a reduction in exacerbations [3]. Controversy continues over whether any of these agents will have a significant impact on symptom relief.

Some non-pharmacologic substances such as hypertonic saline have been found to increase the weight of sputum produced and improve mucociliary clearance in patients with chronic bronchitis. In CF, a number of studies have shown that 7% hypertonic saline was well tolerated and increased the clearance of radioactive particulates, improved lung function, and reduced exacerbations [3]. While not generally recommended or in use, hypertonic saline may prove clinically helpful in specific cases.

Secretions that are thin and copious should raise concerns about oral secretion control and aspiration. While oral secretions are a concern when a tracheotomy is first created, because of changes in upper motor control, over time motor function improves. The improved function translates into less aspiration and less thin, copious secretions. Persistent or worsening of thin secretions should signal a search for causes of swallowing dysfunction.

Humidification

Normal heat and moisture exchange

Ventilation via a tracheotomy eliminates the necessary functions of the nose, including humidification of inspired air. This drier-than-normal air may lead to thickened secretions, interference in mucociliary transport, and frank mucosal damage. The normal respiratory system is made up of a number of structures that include nasal turbinates and mucosa, oropharyngeal mucosa, as well as surfaces of the trachea down to the acinar unit. Our nasal pharyngeal system acts as a natural heat and moisture exchanger and has been extensively studied [5]. Ambient air passes along the nasal–pharyngeal surfaces where it is filtered, heated, and humidified until it is the same body temperature and water saturation as the air already in the alveoli. The point in the airway where this occurs is called the isothermal saturation point or boundary. The location of the isothermal saturation point/boundary varies depending on the depth of respiration and relative humidity of inspired gas. In a normal healthy person, it is located just below the carina [5]. The system is not perfectly efficient, with water and heat being lost as water vapor with each breath. Under normal conditions, this loss amounts to about 250 ml of water and 350 kcal of heat per day [5]. Conditioning of inspired air therefore depends on the volume and composition of inspired gas and the airway's inherent ability to condition it [6]. When the upper airway is bypassed, the isothermal point changes and moves downstream. If there is insufficient water content of inspired gas, it causes damage to the epithelium, loss of ciliary action, thickening of secretions, and change of airway responsiveness to the more proximal airways [7]. Significant heat loss with dry gases used in anesthesia has been described in infants and adults [7].

When discussing humidity, the amount of water content can be expressed as a percentage or absolute concentration. Absolute humidity is the actual volume of water present in a given volume of air and is usually expressed as milligrams of water per liter of air. Relative humidity is expressed as the ratio of water vapor in air to the amount that can maximally exist in air at a set temperature. At 37 °C and 100% relative humidity, alveolar air has 44 mg of water per liter. The use of heated and humidified gases was noted to ameliorate the detrimental airway changes of non-conditioned inspired air and animal and human studies sought to determine optimal humidification levels [7]. The American Association for Respiratory Care Clinical Practice Guidelines recommends that inspired gas contain a minimum of 30 mg of water per liter at 30 °C [8]. Suggested ranges of humidification for a normal airway are 32–34 °C with an inspiratory absolute humidity of 36–40 mg/l.

The intratracheal temperature in tracheotomized patients during inspiration has been directly measured and varies between 28 and 31 °C on inspiration (normal 31–32 °C) and between 32 and 36 °C during expiration (normal 33–36 °C) [9]. Thus, warming of the inspired air should also be considered in the care of these patients.

Methods to humidify air

No one method of humidification is ideal for all patients. A basic understanding of the different methods and their limitations and pitfalls will help match the method chosen for the individual patient. The three broad classifications of humidifiers are: bubble humidifier; passover humidifier; and HME [10]. The amount of humidification a device successfully supplies is very similar to our natural respiratory system and depends on the temperature of the inspired gas and time and amount of surface area that the gas has in contact with the liquid. A bubble humidifier works by passing or "bubbling" air or oxygen through water. By passing the gas through water, water vapor content of the air is raised. As gas flow increases, contact time of the gas with the liquid is reduced, translating into reduced humidification. A passover humidifier system employs the principle of direct contact of the gas by passing over the surface of water, as in a simple reservoir system. To increase the contact surface area, wicks are added. A membrane humidifier allows water vapor molecules to pass through, keeping liquid and pathogens from the airstream. Heating a bubble or passover humidifier system increases the water vapor content of inspired gas by increasing water vapor pressure.

In standard heated humidifier systems, if the temperature in a room is much cooler than the conditioned gas delivered to the patient, condensation in the connection tubing occurs, often referred to as "rain out." The condensate in the tubing poses a number of risks to both the patient and caregiver. Water collected in tubing connected to a patient causes impedance of the gas flow and could be aspirated. As contamination of the circuit by patient flora normally occurs in hours, the condensate becomes contaminated, with increased risk to staff when they remove extraneous fluid. Methods to minimize the effect or development of the

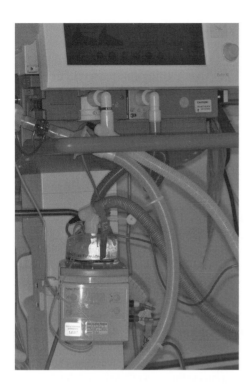

Figure 13.1 Heat and humidification unit on ventilator circuit.

Figure 13.2 Heat Moisture Exchange (HME).

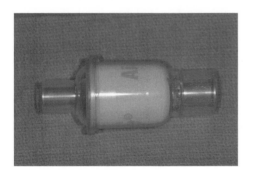

condensate include placement of a water trap in line with the ventilator circuit or use of a heated wire to prevent water condensation. Some authors recommend monitoring of both temperature and humidification because of drying of secretions and mucus plugging when only temperature is monitored (Figure 13.1).

An HME device has been referred to as an "artificial nose." It is a passive system that captures heat and water vapor on exhalation. Claes Allander designed this device in the mid-1950s as a method of humidifying air in patients after tracheotomy. Since then, other devices have been developed and tested for how well they conserve moisture and heat. The design and performance standards are set by the International Organization for Standards and include measures of airway resistance and dead space (Figure 13.2). HMEs are classified into a simple condenser, hygroscopic condenser, or hydrophobic condenser. A simple condenser uses the same principles of heat transfer that occurs when air passes over surfaces. Expired air warms the HME device surfaces and water vapor condenses on it as the vapor contacts the HME's cooler surface. The cooler inspired air is then warmed as it passes through the HME, and water vapor is given up to the drier air. This system is able to capture about 50% of the patient's exhaled moisture. A hygroscopic condenser uses a low thermal conducting element impregnated by a salt that readily absorbs moisture. During exhalation, the water vapor is in contact with cooler surfaces and condenses. The hydroscopic salts directly absorb some of the water content. On inspiration, the salts release the water content back into the air. This system is about 70% efficient. A hydrophobic condenser uses a low thermal conducting element with a large water resistant surface area. The large temperature change on inspiration and exhalation results in greater water condensation available for the next breath. This system is also about 70% efficient in conserving moisture.

The type of humidifier that is used depends on the patient's requirements. HMEs are contraindicated in a number of circumstances, which include secretions that are thick, bloody, and copious. The secretions can clog the HME and increase airway resistance and work of breathing. HMEs are contraindicated when the patient's minute ventilation is high. The efficiency of HME devices is limited by high flows, as the contact time with surfaces within the HME are not sufficient. The HME is also contraindicated if the patient's body temperature is less than 32 °C. In this circumstance, the HME will not warm the patient secondary to similarity to ambient temperature; therefore, external methods to provide heat are recommended. HMEs are also contraindicated when exhaled tidal volumes are less than 70% of delivered volume (i.e., cuffless systems or bronchopleural fistulas). Insufficient volume of air passing both directions through the HME reduces contact time and efficiency of the device.

Some controversy exists in the use of HME devices. The performance specifications of HMEs used to provide humidification during anesthesia do not always match that of the International Standards Organization (ISO) specifications. Studies of the devices in clinical practice have shown that the *in vivo* performance does not always correspond [11]. Other authors have developed simulated clinical models and have noted variable performance between devices [12]. The HME device has also been studied in ventilated patients, where some authors have found an increased work of breathing and impedance, which may hinder weaning [13,14]. HMEs have been associated with gradual reduction of endotracheal tube diameter secondary to blockage by secretions within the tube lumen. Duration of HME use is generally recommended as less than 96 hours of continuous use, but may be less if contraindications develop. Anecdotal use of an HME for more than 96 hours exists but there are no studies to support this.

The need for humidification and type of device preferred should be determined on an individual basis and can be directed by the patient's concerns as well as observation of secretions and trachea mucosal damage, and patient's need for mobility. A patient tethered to a ventilator has the choice of a heated humidification system or an HME. For non-ventilated patients, a humidified tracheotomy collar provides similar results. The mobile patient may find an HME device ("artificial nose") provides adequate moisture, and additionally a filter effect for particulates in the air [15]. Use of HME devices long term is primarily based on individual practice, and is not evidence-based. An ambulatory patient who requires higher humidification would require a portable humidification system. In these cases, the effect of tracheal sprays versus hand-held nebulizers has been investigated with no clear superior device noted. Many clinicians believe that the stable, systemically adequately hydrated adult patient typically will adapt to breathing room air [16]. It is presumed that a new equilibrium is established and compensations made for the new isothermic saturation boundary position [6]. Several authors note this, but no studies have been done to support or refute this observation. Some patients will therefore elect to wear only a cloth or foam bib device to act as filter [17]. Some clinicians advocate complete home humidification, or at least bedroom humidifiers, to aid the mobile tracheotomy patient. Regular care and maintenance of these humidifier units must be done to limit bacterial and fungal growth.

Suctioning

In a normally respiring patient, mucociliary transport provides a large portion of the cleaning of lower airways. This process is significantly augmented by a cough. A cough consists of a deep inspiration, glottic closure, and a forceful exhalation. The glottis opens rapidly after subglottic pressure has built, to create a forceful exhalation that can carry secretions upward and out of the respiratory tract. When the larynx is "bypassed" via tracheotomy, the development of subglottic pressure and rapid release, essential to a good cough, are not possible. Therefore, tracheotomized patients have reduced cough efficiency. Additionally, patients requiring tracheotomy may also have neuromuscular weakness, which further reduces effectiveness of the cough. While some techniques can be helpful to minimize these secretion issues, the key procedure to reduce mucus plugging and assist in clearing secretions is suctioning. Suctioning provides the added assistance in clearing secretions not cleared by the ineffectual cough. The three main controversies in suctioning involve routine suctioning versus as needed, closed versus open suction systems, and instillation of normal saline when suctioning.

Risks of suctioning

Suctioning via the tracheotomy provides mechanical clearing of secretions from the lower airway but can also traumatize airway mucosa. This technique requires the introduction of a foreign body to the airway, as well as a suctioning force. Animal studies have shown both mucosal inflammation and trauma related to suction catheters that corresponded to clinical guidelines and circumstances similar to clinical care [18]. This inflammation is induced in part by catheter coming into physical contact with the mucosa. Typically, this injury is microscopic. The suction force created through the catheter grossly injures the mucosa in a very short contact time. Direct suction force on the mucosa can cause loss of the mucosal epithelium, as well as inflammation and hemorrhage in the submucosal tissues. The greater the suction force or the more frequent the suctioning, the greater the damage seen [18]. Multi-eyed catheters are felt to reduce trauma as compared with single eyelet catheters because suction trauma is directly related to strength of the contacted suction force. Secondary eyelets are present on multiple planes, so that at any moment, if some of the eyelets are in contact with the tracheal mucosa, others are not. These off-plane eyelets allow for airflow through the secondary eyelets when another eyelet is in direct contact with mucosa, reducing suction pressure at the level of the mucosa. Thus, these secondary eyelets serve as "release valves" for the suction force to reduce injury (Figure 13.3). Direct mucosal injury can be minimized by adopting a "shallow suctioning" technique, where the suction catheter is only introduced to the end of the tracheotomy tube itself, and not into the trachea proper [19]. Secretions transported or coughed up the tracheotomy tube are thus removed, but damage is minimized by reduced contact with mucosa. Another notable observation is the reduction in mucociliary transport velocity, and thus the inherent clearing mechanism,

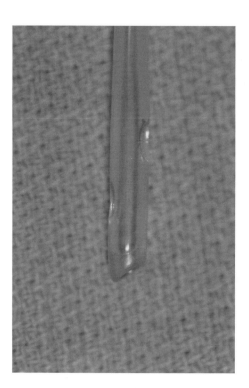

Figure 13.3 Suction catheter tip demonstrating multiple eyelets, off plane from each other.

created transiently after suctioning with even the multi-eyelet catheters [20]. Additionally, pain and hemodynamic changes are encountered during suctioning in ICU patients [21]. While most patients rate suctioning as a mild pain, almost half report moderate to severe pain scores. Given all of these factors, if routine suctioning is instituted, then potentially unnecessary airway trauma and pain are inflicted on the patient. Furthermore, suctioning may cause airway collapse and alveolar derecruitment. This is particularly significant in the pediatric patient with their lower lung volume, and pulmonary reserve. Therefore, recommendations for suctioning are primarily based on clinically necessity individualized to patient factors, including secretion viscosity and volume, quality of cough reflex, and neuromuscular status (baseline and iatrogenic weakness) [15] and not a routine schedule [8]. Oral suctioning of secretions in a patient who cannot manage them effectively is also advisable to reduce the potential aspiration.

Open versus closed suctioning systems

The decision to use open versus closed suctioning systems predominantly involve the artificially ventilated patient, although closed systems are available for spontaneously breathing tracheotomized patients (Figures 13.4 and 13.5). A closed system has an adapter that allows the introduction of the suction catheter into the airway, without disconnecting the ventilator circuit, or even direct hand contact with the catheter. The catheter is covered by a plastic sheath when not in use within the airway, and has a finger-operated valve to turn the suction on and off. This is in contrast to the open system, which requires disconnecting the ventilator circuit to allow the introduction of a catheter via clean versus sterile

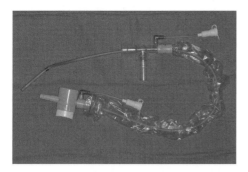

Figure 13.4 Closed suction catheter system.

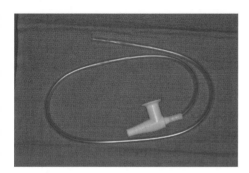

Figure 13.5 Open suction catheter system.

technique (see Wound care section below). During this suctioning period, the patient is not receiving ventilator support. While pre-suctioning hyperventilation and hyperoxygenation are typically performed, the open system significantly disrupts ventilation. The purported benefits of the closed system for ventilated patients are in improved oxygenation during suctioning and reduction of ventilator-associated pneumonia (VAP). As the patient does not need to be taken off the ventilator circuit with the closed system, there is less respiratory physiologic disturbance. Most studies investigating this issue were done on endotracheal-intubated patients that differ from the chronic tracheotomized patient. However, some similarities exist and can be generalized. Closed suctioning systems have benefits for ventilated patients, including less arterial and venous oxygen desaturation and lower costs per patient than open systems [22]. However, for the non-ventilated, mobile tracheotomy patient, an open system is much more practical. In regards to VAP and differences between open and closed systems, the literature is contradictory. While logically a closed system may seem less likely to be contaminated and thus seed the lower airway (e.g., "hands-off technique"), there are no consistent patterns showing reduced infection rates between these two techniques [22].

Normal saline instillation

The use of normal saline instillation (NSI) during suctioning has been more extensively researched. NSI had been traditionally taught as a routine necessity in ventilated patients via endotracheal tube or tracheotomy. The thought process in using normal saline was that it loosens secretions, achieves a bronchial lavage, lubricates the suction catheter, and stimulates cough. While it clearly does achieve the latter, the remainder of the claims is less clear. Studies have shown that little of the saline ever reached the lung periphery, defeating the idea of bronchoalveolar lavage. Oxygenation may be adversely effected by NSI. Several studies show little difference in oxygenation whether NSI is used or not, but some do indeed show greater desaturation with NSI use. Thus, NSI is felt to have no or an adverse effect on oxygenation. Concern exists regarding infections of the lower airway with NSI. Observational studies have shown that contamination of saline by personnel while opening the vial before instillation is not uncommon. Laboratory studies have shown NSI also dislodges a greater number of bacteria that colonize the endotracheal or tracheotomy tube by 48 hours than suction catheter placement alone, thus potentially increasing the chance of lower airway infection [23]. Summarizing, NSI has no supported benefits in the literature, and several concerns regarding detriment, and therefore, NSI cannot be recommended as standard practice for care.

Sterile versus clean technique

Traditionally, the suctioning of tracheotomy tubes was felt to require sterile technique, and this idea often is still taught in nursing and respiratory therapy training. While sterile practices would appear to be obviously superior to clean techniques, most authorities now favor good clean technique as opposed to sterility. As with open versus closed suction systems, the rate of airway infection is not statistically greater in clean technique care. Additionally, observational studies show that compliance with sterile technique is poor among nurses, and that emphasis on clean technique allowed greater consistency than attempts at complete sterility [24]. Patients are unlikely to be willing or able to adhere to sterile technique in a home setting. Self-suctioning, or caring for a family member's tracheotomy can be stressful, and to add sterility to the process may create hesitancy or even promote passive neglect, subsequently increasing potential morbidity. Clean technique has been shown to induce no greater rate of respiratory infection than sterile technique and, therefore, is recommended practice in general for tracheotomy care. In ventilated patients, the closed suction systems aid in maintaining this clean technique versus open suction, yet largely the infection rates do not differ [22].

Wound management

Unlike many surgical wounds, a tracheotomy involves the creation of the wound with planned healing by secondary intention. Given that management of this particular wound can also impact on respiration, particular care is needed in the postoperative period until the wound is well healed. Dislodgement of the tracheotomy tube before establishment of a defined tract can have tragic consequences. While these issues are covered in chapters about the surgery itself, wound management deserves a review given that many patients are transferred from the institution where the original tracheotomy was placed to other institutions. With increased pressure from healthcare payers to reduce length of hospital stays, on occasion, this transfer may even occur before the first tracheotomy tube change.

Initial tube exchange

Based on tradition and local practices, most surgeons and healthcare providers feel the surgical team who performed the procedure should do the first tracheotomy tube change. One of the presumed purposes of this change is to assess the tract for healing. Tracheotomy tracts will epithelialize, creating a tracheocutaneous tract. Several factors may adversely affect this healing, including factors affecting healing in general (e.g., chemotherapy agents, steroids, diabetes, vascular disease). Additional local factors may also play a role. The larger the wound, the greater the time is for healing via secondary intention. This size issue may be in terms of the linear size of the incision, the degree of surrounding tissue dissection, or the depth of the tract (i.e., patient with thick neck tissues). Therefore, obese patients face a particular challenge, as wider access may be needed for initial visualization during surgical placement, and the wound is deeper related to subcutaneous adipose tissue. Additionally, moderately vascularized tissues, such as adipose tissue, require greater healing times and are more vulnerable to infection. Infection in the proximity of the surgical wound can lengthen healing times and stoma maturity in all patients. Additional local factors, which may adversely affect healing, include radiation and tissue ischemia or necrosis secondary to local trauma of surgery. The potential for placing the tracheotomy tube into a false passage is higher until this tract is sufficiently healed to resist the typical force used in an exchange. The surgeon can assess the degree of wound healing during that first tube change and plan for the most appropriate personnel and timing to safely perform future changes.

Another reason for the tracheotomy tube to be changed at 1 week by the surgeon involves reducing infection. The thought process is that the initial tracheotomy tube is placed in an open wound environment and may become contaminated. Exchanging the tube may provide a reduced reservoir for infection. Neither of these rationales is supported by the scientific literature. While it may seem prudent for the surgical team to change the tube initially to assess healing, and to determine if the tract is sufficiently developed to allow for transfer or tube changes by other personnel, the necessity of this is not supported by current evidence. The timing of the initial change is also a point of controversy. Limited scientific literature is available to define proper timing for this change. While some studies in the pediatric otolaryngology community support early changes at day 3, most surgeons seem to favor a 3–7-day time frame [25]. Particular nuances of the patient's clinical status may alter the timing. Some case reports describe the tragic loss of airway in this early period. Loss of airway is most likely during initial tract development, and therefore, the practice of changing the tube early may create additional risk, without scientifically proven merit.

Granulation tissue

There is some support in the literature for frequent routine tracheotomy tube changes after placement, in an effort to reduce granulation tissue. The tube is felt to serve as a reservoir for bacteria and biofilms, and thus regular changes may reduce local and respiratory infections. Granulation tissue, a polypoid inflammatory vascular tissue, may form in the peristomal or suprastomal area. Infection, reflux, inflammation from sutures, and even surgical glove powder has been implicated in granulation formation [26]. Tracheotomy tube change then may serve to decrease the rate of infection. Yaremchuk [26] demonstrated a significant reduction in granulation formation requiring surgical intervention when the tracheotomy tube was routinely changed every 2 weeks.

Granulation tissue may interfere with tracheotomy tube changes, block the airway, limit phonation, bleed, or contribute to local peristomal moisture and skin maceration issues. While prevention is foremost, granulation incidence is quite high and cited to be between 10% and 80%. The position of the tube in the tracheotomy site needs to be noted as proper fitting devices reduce long-term issues such as granulation tissue formation. The scientific data supporting a particular modality of therapy for granulations are lacking. Suggested treatments for peristomal granulations include: steroid creams, antibiotic creams, silver nitrate or electrocautery, and polyurethane foam dressings. In the case of tracheal granulations, inhaled steroid, bronchoscopic resection with laser or resectoscope, and trans-stomal resection with bronchoscopic guidance have been described [26]. Some patients are chronically plagued with recurrent granulations, while others may never experience issues despite long-term tracheotomy; therefore, practices may be individualized according to the patient and local practices until there are evidence-based studies to support a particular protocol.

Wound care and cleaning

The tracheotomy site needs to be monitored for a wide range of problems, including site integrity, presence of secretions, and type of drainage, if any. The tracheotomy site cleaning methods and dressings are variable among practitioners. Local care agents used for cleaning the site include hydrogen peroxide, soap and water, medical disinfectants, and dilute acetic acid. None of these materials have been shown to be beneficial or superior in a scientific manner. In many cases, the regimen may be influenced by insurance reimbursement for supplies, similarly not based on scientific principle [16] (Figures 13.6–13.8). In addition,

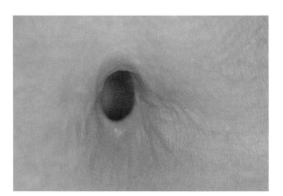

Figure 13.6 Well-healed healthy tracheotomy stoma.

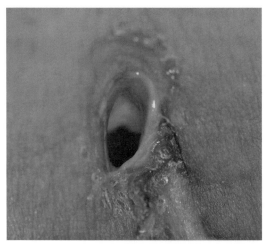

Figure 13.7 Healed, moderately healthy tracheotomy stoma, with some secretions and granulations.

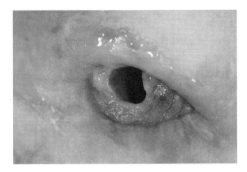

Figure 13.8 Healed, but unhealthy tracheotomy stoma, with prominent secretions and granulations.

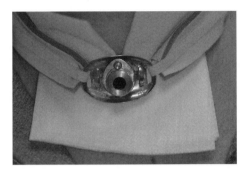

Figure 13.9 Metal tracheotomy tube with gauze dressing.

dressings appear primarily driven by local practices and patient preference. The purpose of dressings is to absorb secretions from around the tracheotomy tube, or from the tube lumen. Additionally, granulation tissue around the stoma site may produce exudates and thus create a local moist environment. Poor secretion control can create peristomal maceration and inflammation. The materials used for these dressings may include typical surgical gauze, gauze drain sponges, or foam sponges. The latter two typically come with a fenestration or slit to allow placement around the tracheotomy tube. Surgical gauze is generally made from woven 100% cotton, while drain sponges are made of non-woven, polyester/rayon blends (Figure 13.9). Foam sponges are more absorbent, and may provide greater protection from excoriation from tracheotomy tube flanges. Gauzes and sponges manufactured with slits or cutouts may be better than cut cotton gauze, as the latter may form lint fragments. Some research supports the use of antimicrobial impregnated drain sponges to reduce pathogenic organisms around the stoma, while less dramatically affecting normal skin flora, important to helping maintain skin barrier function [27].

As the tracheotomy tube is a manufactured medical device, it has a finite lifespan and a rate of failure. Therefore, the tracheotomy tube needs to be constantly monitored for damage or failure and changed, if found. Common issues include cuff failure and leak, damage to the monitoring balloon in cuffed tubes, cracked inner or outer cannulas, or failure of the external flange-shaft joint. Routine changes should be planned in such a fashion to avoid these failures. However, in unexpected events, rapid intervention may be necessary to ensure adequate ventilation, or to prevent aspiration and a potential airway foreign body.

Conclusions

- Normal tracheal secretions must be managed, and efforts made to reduce excessive secretions in tracheotomy patients.

- Maintenance of humidity and heat for these patients is beneficial in reducing damage to the lower respiratory mucosa.

- Suctioning is a key procedure. It can aid many tracheotomy patients in clearing secretions. However, routine use of suctioning is not recommended, but rather when needed at sensible intervals is best.

- Saline instillation when suctioning is controversial and generally not supported by the literature.

- Tracheotomy wound care is performed in an effort to minimize local complications, including infection and granulations. Multiple techniques have been recommended for treatment of granulations, with none singled out in the literature as best.

- Routine tracheotomy tube changes may aid in reducing granulation tissue formation, and possible device failures, which could negatively impact the patient.

Returning to the initial case presentation, the following questions came to mind. Should his home routine be maintained? What problems might be encountered? What are the options of care?

If secretions are easily mobilized by his own cough and clearance techniques, less intervention may be better, and his routine may be maintained. If he has difficulty clearing secretions, use of therapies to augment secretion removal can be tried. If there is crusting or thickening of secretions, the HME device becomes relatively contraindicated, and a heated humidifier system should be used instead.

References

1. Rogers DF. Physiology of airway mucus secretion and pathophysiology of hypersecretion.*Respir Care* 2007; **52**(9): 1134–46; discussion 1146–9.

2. Voynow JA, Rubin BK. Mucins, mucus, and sputum. *Chest* 2009; **135**(2): 505–12.

3. Rogers DF. Mucoactive agents for airway mucus hypersecretory diseases. *Respir Care* 2007; **52**(9): 1176–93; discussion 1193–7.

4. King M. Experimental models for studying mucociliary clearance. *Eur Respir J* 1998; **11**: 222–8.

5. Walker, Wells RE Jr., Merrill EW. Heat and water exchange in the respiratory tract. *Am J Med* 1961; **30**: 259–67.

6. Shelly MP, Lloyd GM, Park GR. A review of the mechanisms and methods of humidification of inspired gases. *Intensive Care Med* 1988; **14**: 1–9.

7. Chalon J, Loew DA, Malebranche J. Effects of dry anesthetic gases on tracheobronchial ciliated epithelium. *Anesthesiology* 1972; **37**(3): 338–43.

8. AARC Clinical Practice Guideline. Endotracheal suctioning of mechanically ventilated adults and children with artificial airways. American Association for Respiratory Care. *Respir Care* 1993; **38**(5): 500–4.

9. Liener K, Durr J, Leiacker R, Rozsasi A, Keck T. Measurement of tracheal humidity and temperature. *Respiration* 2006; **73**(3): 324–8.

10. Fink J. Humidity and bland aerosol therapy. In: R Kacmarek, RL Wilkins, JK Stoller, editors. *Egan's Fundamentals of Respiratory Care*, 9th edn. St. Louis, Missouri: Mosby Elselvier, 2009; 775–90.

11. Lemmens HJ, Brock-Utne JG. Heat and moisture exchange devices: are they doing what they are supposed to do? *Anesth Analg* 2004; **98**(2): 382–5, table of contents.

12. Unal N, Kanhai JK, Buijk SL, *et al.* A novel method of evaluation of three heat-moisture exchangers in six different ventilator settings. *Intensive Care Med* 1998; **24**(2): 138–46.

13. Girault C, Breton L, Richard JC, *et al.* Mechanical effects of airway humidification devices in difficult to wean patients. *Crit Care Med* 2003; **31**(5): 1306–11.

14. Le Bourdelles G, Mier L, Fiquet B, *et al.* Comparison of the effects of heat and moisture exchangers and heated humidifiers on ventilation and gas exchange during weaning trials from mechanical ventilation. *Chest* 1996; **110**(5): 1294–8.

15. De Leyn P, Bedert L, Delcroix M, *et al.* Tracheotomy: clinical review and guidelines. *Eur J Cardiothorac Surg* 2007; **32**(3): 412–21.

16. Lewarski JS. Long-term care of the patient with a tracheostomy. *Respir Care* 2005; **50**(4): 534–7.

17. Wright SE, VanDahm K. Long-term care of the tracheostomy patient. *Clin Chest Med* 2003; **24**(3): 473–87.

18. Sackner MA, Landa JF, Greeneltch N, Robinson MJ. Pathogenesis and prevention of tracheobronchial damage with suction procedures. *Chest* 1973; **64**(3): 284–90.

19. Sherman JM, Davis S, Albamonte-Petrick S, *et al.* Care of the child with a chronic tracheostomy. This official statement of the American Thoracic Society was adopted by the ATS Board of Directors, July 1999. *Am J Respir Crit Care Med* 2000; **161**: 297–308.

20. Landa JF, Kwoka MA, Chapman GA, Brito M, Sackner MA. Effects of suctioning on mucociliary transport. *Chest* 1980; **77**(2): 202–7.

21. Arroyo-Novoa CM, Figueroa-Ramos MI, Puntillo KA, *et al.* Pain related to tracheal suctioning in awake acutely and critically ill adults: a descriptive study. *Intensive Crit Care Nurs* 2008; **24**: 20–7.

22. Johnson KL, Kearney PA, Johnson SB, *et al.* Closed versus open endotracheal suctioning: costs and physiologic consequences. *Crit Care Med* 1994; **22**(4): 658–66.

23. Ackerman MH, Ecklund MM, Abu-Jumah M. A review of normal saline instillation: implications for practice. *Dimens Crit Care Nurs* 1996; **15**: 31–8.

24. Harris RB, Hyman RB. Clean vs. sterile tracheotomy care and level of pulmonary infection. *Nurs Res* 1984; **33**(2): 80–5.

25. Tabaee A, Lando T, Rickert S, Stewart MG, Kuhel WI. Practice patterns, safety, and rationale for tracheostomy tube changes: a survey of otolaryngology training programs. *Laryngoscope* 2007; **117**(4): 573–6.

26. Yaremchuk K. Regular tracheostomy tube changes to prevent formation of granulation tissue. *Laryngoscope* 2003; **113**: 1–10.

27. Motta GJ, Trigilia D. The effect of an antimicrobial drain sponge dressing on specific bacterial isolates at tracheostomy sites. *Ostomy Wound Manage* 2005; **51**: 60–2, 64–6.

Tracheotomy education for home care

Jodie E. Landis, Michael K. Hurst, and Brian W. Grose

Case presentation

John is a 27-year-old man who was involved in a car accident. Injuries included cervical fractures (C2, C3) right broken tibia, multiple broken ribs, punctured right lung, with other minor injuries. Because of his injuries, John is quadriplegic and he had a tracheotomy placed early in his hospitalization. He was discharged from the hospital to inpatient rehabilitation. John is very fortunate that he has a supportive family, including a wife, parents, and one sibling. Training to manage John's tracheotomy began in hospital and continued at the rehabilitation facility.

Tracheotomy education

People typically are overwhelmed when they are informed that a tracheotomy is in their future. A tracheotomy is typically the result of a more ominous medical diagnosis and other risks and complications may initially be given a higher priority than the tracheotomy. The long-term implications of having a tracheotomy are often not fully considered until the patient is home where s/he finally begins to grasp the procedure fully. Frequently asked questions are "Will I still be able to eat?," "Will I be able to talk?," "Will I ever be able to leave my home or go on vacation?" The answer to all of these questions is yes; however, to be successful, comprehensive education and training are necessary for people to manage a tracheotomy at home over the long term. There are few reliable controlled studies involving the standard of care for outpatient tracheotomies. This may be due to the variability among patient's physical and cognitive abilities and as well as the variety of available tracheotomies.

Many patients and their families find themselves at home feeling unsure of what to do to maintain even an adequate health status. To care adequately for a tracheotomy, there are four basic categories of skills that must be learned: suctioning; tracheotomy changes; caring for stoma and surrounding skin; and emergency skills. This chapter will discuss basic guidelines for patient and caregiver education in all four of these areas, in addition to the professional's responsibility.

Education should begin as soon as possible, ideally before the surgery. Many tracheotomy patients require additional support to assist in managing tracheotomies, especially during the period immediately following their discharge from the hospital. This support must reach beyond medical professionals within the hospital to include the patient and their family, friends, or other support network. At discharge, patients may have been well trained and

Tracheotomy Management: A Multidisciplinary Approach, ed. Peggy A. Seidman, David Goldenberg and Elizabeth H. Sinz. Published by Cambridge University Press.

educated; however, they have always had the support of medical personnel to assist with troubleshooting when difficulties occurred. Going home may be a daunting task for many patients and their families, particularly for those with young children. The multidisciplinary team should safely prepare and plan for patients to return to their home environment with a coordinated and individualized plan. One successful approach is to arrange a meeting (i.e., before discharge) with key participants, including the patient, primary caregivers, physician, social worker, respite care representative, home health providers, speech language pathologist (SLP), and respiratory therapist. These individuals play a key role in the success of a tracheotomized patient's recovery.

The physician who placed the tracheotomy is responsible for insuring that adequate training for the patient and caregivers is completed. They should be accessible to the patient to answer any questions that may arise after the patient has gone home. The physician should also establish a plan to follow the progress of the patient and to determine possible decannulation. This plan should be conveyed to the patient in clear and concise terms during the multidisciplinary meeting to establish clearly each individual's role in the recovery process.

The social worker's role is to provide the patient and family with information on medical coverage and additional avenues available to expand coverage if necessary. Discharge planning is also completed by the social worker, ensuring all details have been addressed for the patient's return home. Occasionally, patients have difficulty dealing with the emotions involved following the placement of a tracheotomy. A social worker has the capabilities to direct the patient to the appropriate support groups or professionals to assist in handling these emotions.

Respite workers are available for primary caregivers to provide a break from the continuous responsibilities these patients require. Primary caregivers must ensure that respite workers are properly trained in every aspect of a patient's daily care and medical needs. It is the respite workers' responsibility to assist in completion of everyday activities in their entirety, from suctioning and tracheotomy cleaning to leisure activities and meal preparation.

Home health providers are available for support and to answer questions, and may be a caregiver and patient's most readily available source of information since they are in the home on a regular basis. Frequently, these individuals are nurses addressing any problems that the patient and primary caregivers are experiencing. Home health services are available to discharged patients who meet specific established insurance requirements for skilled assistance, which generally include the following:

(1) The patient must require "skilled" services in the home environment. That means the patient continues to require the care of a professional to meet some or all of the needs. Professionals include speech therapy, physical therapy, occupational therapy, and nursing to assist patients in resuming independence. Each qualifying service will assess the patient to determine need and frequency of visitations based upon physical status. A plan will then be developed with goals established for the patient to achieve.

(2) The patient must be followed up by a physician who will agree and sign the goals and finally generate orders. This step is required for the home healthcare provider to be reimbursed for the provided service.

(3) The patient must be considered "homebound." The term homebound has exceptions that allow for infrequent trips, but the patient is not permitted to drive.

SLPs play an important role in a tracheotomized patient's ability to regain independence. For the initial period after a tracheotomy is placed, the patient is unable to speak and must

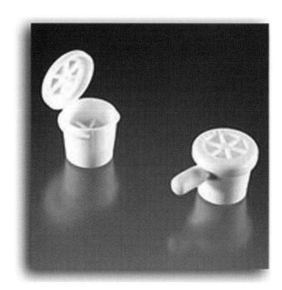

Figure 14.1 Phonate speaking valve.

communicate with individuals in his environment via an alternative means (writing, picture board, hand signals). Upon a referral from the patient's physician, an SLP assists the patient in utilizing a speaking valve that aids the patient in verbally conveying wants and needs. Speaking valves open during inhalation and close on exhalation allowing the patient to speak by redirecting exhaled air through the vocal folds. This allows the person to have a natural voice. Speaking valves must be worn on cuffless or deflated cuffed tracheotomies, otherwise the exhaled air cannot be expelled, creating a dangerous situation. If the patient has been assessed and muscles of the larynx and pharynx are functionally intact, all secretions are expelled through the oral cavity. This decreases the need for suctioning and helps prevent skin breakdown around the stoma site. The most common type of speaking valve utilized is the "Passy–Muir" valve. Other types of speaking valves include the Phonate Speaking Valve (Figure 14.1) and the Shikani French Speaking Valve.

Difficulty eating shortly after placement of a tracheotomy is common, and indicates a referral to an SLP. Typical signs that a referral would be beneficial include frequent coughing during meals, sensation of food lodged in the esophagus, and frequent respiratory infection. The SLP, in conjunction with a radiologist, can perform a test specifically to examine the muscles related to the swallow and overall function to determine cause of problem. The specific test performed will depend upon the patient's functioning level. Alert patients with limited muscular impairment may participate in a modified barium swallow study. During this study, the patient is presented with barium in different consistencies by the SLP. The radiologist observes the flow of the barium insuring that no foreign material is entering into the lungs during the swallow. Fiberoptic endoscopic examination of swallowing may be used when there are serious concerns about aspiration, making a modified barium swallow study ill advised.

All of these previously mentioned topics were presented to the case study individual, John (tracheotomized patient). John was very fortunate that he was at a site that coordinated the multiple specialties, including physicians and therapists. He was closely followed by his otolaryngologist-head and neck surgeon with referral to appropriate specialties. After John was taken off the vent, he was referred to the SLP for a swallow evaluation. John remained alert,

Table 14.1 Recommendations for disposable and non-disposable equipment typically needed by patients upon returning home from the hospital following tracheotomy.

Non-disposable items	Disposable items
Suction pump	Suction catheters
Portable suction (internal battery)	Suction tubing
Nebulizer (portable)	Nebulizer tubing and reservoir
Tracheal dilators	Tracheotomy mask
Cuff pressure – manometer	Spare tracheotomy tubes (including smaller sizes as an alternative)
Trach mask	Velcro holder/ribbon ties
	Heat moisture exchanger
	Tracheotomy cleaning kit supplies
	Stoma dressings
	Stoma protectors

Adapted from Russell and Matta [1].

oriented, and cooperative during the modified barium swallow study. The results of the study indicated decreased laryngeal elevation resulting in food and liquids spilling into the airway (aspiration). The recommendation made by the SLP was for alternative means of nutrition be provided (gastric tube – G tube) until the laryngeal muscles could be restored to a functional status. A Passy–Muir speaking valve was also recommended secondary to John's stable respiratory status to increase his ability to communicate. A social worker was assigned to John to assist him in developing a plan for completing medical tasks at home. The social worker synchronized family members' schedules for "hands-on" training of tracheotomy care. In addition, home health providers were established to stay with John while his wife was at work during the day. All home equipment and supplier's information was provided by the social worker.

Equipment requirements for home care

Mechanical and disposable equipment needs should be established and placed in the home environment before the person leaves hospital. Table 14.1 lists recommendations for disposable and non-disposable equipment typically needed by patients upon returning home from the hospital following tracheotomy. It is recommended that a patient have at least a 7-day supply of disposable materials.

Additional items that are optional but assist in optimizing efficiency include the following:

- Resuscitation bag
- Stethoscope
- Monitor
- Thermometer
- Room humidifier

Most patients require about 4–6 weeks to integrate fully into normal activities of daily living after being discharged from hospital. Because the normal anatomy has changed, specialized equipment may be needed to assist in completing these activities successfully and safely. Despite good planning, unanticipated situations can still arise. The following additional items are often useful in the basic management of tracheotomies:

(1) Stoma shields are very helpful in providing protection to the airway and lungs. Individuals must be careful not to inhale foreign particles as the body no longer has a natural filtering mechanism for the air that is inhaled now that the nose has been bypassed. Dust, aerosol, and powder can be highly dangerous for a patient with a tracheotomy. Stoma shields act as a filter preventing these particles from entering the stoma and leading to a possible respiratory irritation or infection. The shields come in a variety of sizes and materials. Some patients choose not to purchase commercially produced shields, but to create their own via scarves or other individualized preferences.

(2) A humidification collar may be necessary. With the placement of a tracheotomy and bypassing the nasal cavity for airflow, the body no longer is capable of providing warmth or moisture to the inhaled air. Without this ability, mucus may become thick and hazardous to the patient. Thick, increased mucus production tends to result in difficulty obtaining adequate oxygenation and ventilation. A humidification collar is placed over the tracheotomy providing moisture to the air, helping to keep secretions thinner and avoiding mucus plugs. A heat and moisture exchanger may be attached to the inner cannula allowing the patient to be mobile, decreasing the need for humidified air.

(3) Tracheotomy guards are typically designed for the pediatric population to assist in preventing occlusion of the tracheotomy opening. Young children have shortened necks and limited head control, which increases the risk of the tracheotomy becoming occluded. The guard will also help keep articles of clothing and bedding from blocking the airflow through the tracheotomy. The Tilson Trach Guard (Figure 14.2) produced by Beevers Manufacturing (McMinnville, OR, USA) is an example of this item.

(4) Shower shields can be fabricated from a variety of waterproof materials to keep water from running into the tracheotomy during a shower. These shields are reusable and

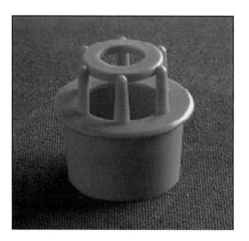

Figure 14.2 Tilson Trach Guard.

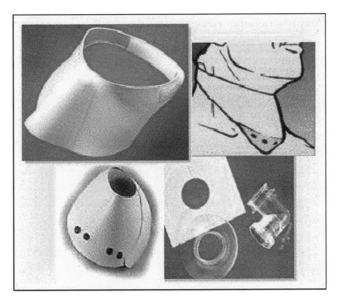

Figure 14.3 Shower shields.

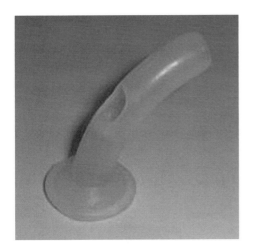

Figure 14.4 Bath Trach.

attach with a velcro strap to make application easy and time efficient. Although these shields are effective for use in the shower, they are not appropriate for swimming. Bath tracheotomies are fenestrated and protect the airway by plugging the stoma. Thin layers of plastic are then applied over the site for additional protection.

Swimming is not usually recommended, especially for children, due to possible leakage around the tracheotomy leading to increased risk of infection and drowning, but it is possible. Overall, physical functioning plays a large role, with cognitive functioning a close second in determining if swimming is an appropriate and safe activity for an individual. If swimming is deemed safe, specialized equipment may be obtained that occludes the stoma and redirects the airflow through the oral cavity. This device is not the same as a speaking valve and it is highly recommended that a suction machine be available in case water enters the airway and causes respiratory distress.

Patient and caregiver guidelines to tracheotomy care

If training takes place before placement of the tracheotomy, the individual and potential caregivers have time to become acquainted with specific techniques demonstrated. Initially education should include basic anatomy, so that individuals can understand appropriate placement during changes and reinsertion of tubing, why talking is difficult, and why humidification is important. Warning signs that may lead to serious complications such as upper airway distress, infection surrounding the stoma, and suspected aspiration should be included as part of the educational process. These are all important issues that must be addressed to increase a patient's independence in a home environment.

The tracheotomy provides a direct window into the airway and lungs; therefore, daily care is required to maintain a healthy respiratory tract. The frequency of care depends upon the patient and the overseeing physician's philosophy on proper management. The minimum recommendations are one time per day tracheotomy and stoma cleaning with tube changes occurring as infrequently as once a month. Factors, including recent placement and increased secretions, typically result in a need for increased frequency of cleaning. Excessive secretions typically lead to skin breakdown, which can lead to infection.

Typical cleaning instructions

Easiest cleaning and maintenance is typically established by developing a routine. Certain standards are recommended for maintaining a clean environment to avoid contaminating the equipment resulting in possible infection of the airway or lungs. The exact approach may vary but, generally, patients should aim for "clean" standards. Thoroughly wash hands and equipment with soap and warm water. To initiate the cleaning process all necessary supplies should be obtained and placed in an easily accessible location before the beginning of tracheotomy care. The patient should lie in the most comfortable position allowable with his neck entirely exposed. If the patient is agitated or excessively irritated it is not recommended that tracheotomy cleaning be completed. Each cleaning should begin with a thorough inspection of the stoma site, looking for any irregularities. Typical symptoms to be aware of include redness or inflammation, pain or soreness, and any discharge or unusual odor. These signs may be indications of a much more serious condition and if they persist, it is recommended that the patient contact a physician.

After inspection of the stoma, clean the stoma and the tube of the tracheotomy. Clean the stoma using sterile technique to prepare and drape the stoma. Hydrogen peroxide and sterile water are used to clean around the stoma and moving outward. Allow the site to dry and place a dressing under the tracheotomy tube. While cleaning the inner cannula soak in hydrogen peroxide. Clean thoroughly with a brush inside and outside then rinse with sterile water. Suction the outer cannula if needed. Then dry the inner cannula and reinsert into the outer cannula and lock into place.

These are not detailed, all-inclusive, instructions for cleaning a stoma site or the inner cannula. Different sources may recommend different procedural techniques and methods for completing these tasks. This is why the physician is responsible for ensuring education and training has taken place before discharge, in an attempt to avoid confusion on the part of the patient.

Tracheotomy kits are available through medical suppliers that ensure cleanliness and provide added convenience. These kits are costly and not always covered by insurance, making it difficult for patients to use them on a daily basis.

Table 14.2 Basic commercial kit

Cotton tipped applicators (Q-tips)
Gloves
Tracheotomy dressing
4 × 4 gauze sponges, unfilled gauze
Tracheotomy ties
Cleaning brush
Hydrogen peroxide
Sterile water

Table 14.3 Basic steps towards stoma cleaning/maintenance

1. Wash hands
2. Position patient
3. Open supplies: Q tips, gauze
4. Fill one cup with hydrogen peroxide and second cup with sterile water
5. Place Q tips in hydrogen peroxide and in water
6. Using the hydrogen peroxide soaked Q tips – work from the stoma outwards to prevent any liquid from entering the airway
7. Using the sterile water soaked Q tip – rinse the area
8. Pat dry with gauze
9. Change the tracheotomy ties and check the skin to make sure no irritation is occurring
10. If needed, place dressing under each wing of the tube

The following are general guidelines to cleaning and maintaining a patient's tracheotomy and the procedure may vary depending upon the patient's physical conditions or other limiting factors.

If the tracheotomy has an inner cannula, this also needs to be cleaned. The inner cannula is the inner portion of the tracheotomy, and may be replacing the obturator.

Basic procedural steps for cleaning the inner cannula:

(1) Wash hands.

(2) Unlock and remove the inner cannula.

(3) Place cannula into hydrogen peroxide and soak for an adequate amount of time (approximately 1 min).

(4) Use brush to clean both inside and outside of the cannula.

Table 14.4 Materials needed

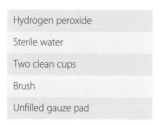

Hydrogen peroxide
Sterile water
Two clean cups
Brush
Unfilled gauze pad

(5) Place cannula into sterile water, soak, and rinse.

(6) Suction the outer cannula if necessary.

(7) Remove inner cannula from water and dry off excess water with gauze pad.

(8) Replace inner cannula making sure it is locked into place.

Suctioning

Suctioning to remove excess secretions and mucus is another important aspect of managing a tracheotomy. There are three main types of suctioning: shallow; premeasured; and deep. Shallow suctioning is the removal of secretions that have already been expelled from the lungs via a cough and are resting in the opening of the tracheotomy. The premeasured technique for suctioning is defined as the insertion of the suction catheter to a predetermined depth that is equivalent to the length of the tracheotomy tube used by the patient. Deep suctioning is considered the insertion of the suction catheter until resistance is met. Much research regarding this method of suctioning indicates that significant tissue damage is generated when deep suctioning is repeatedly implemented to clear secretions. The most frequently utilized technique is premeasured, which is less invasive and as effective for the removal of normal secretion productions. Premeasured catheters are available to increase effectiveness and time efficiency.

Suctioning is typically required when a patient is unable to expel mucus and secretions from lungs by coughing. The frequency of suctioning is highly dependent upon the individual. A minimum of twice daily, once in the morning, and once in the evening is recommended to assess secretions for any possible infection. Three different standards, sterile, modified sterile, and clean, have been established to decrease exposure to infections during suctioning. Sterile technique is the most common method utilized while the patient is still hospitalized and requires the use of a sterile catheter and gloves for each suctioning procedure. The modified sterile technique is the use of a sterile catheter with freshly washed, clean hands, or non-sterile gloved hands for the suctioning procedure. A clean technique is the one most typically implemented by a tracheotomized patient at home. It is the process of using a clean catheter and freshly washed, clean hands or non-sterile gloves for the procedure. Care is taken not to allow the portion of the catheter that will be inserted in the tracheotomy tube to contact any unclean surface.

A general and condensed procedure for suctioning a tracheotomized patient has been outlined below. Materials necessary include suction machine and tubing, suction catheter,

Table 14.5 Procedure for suctioning

1. Obtain suction machine and attach tubing.

2. Place sterile water in bowl and set to side.

3. Wash hands and put on gloves.

4. Remove suction catheter from package and attach to suction tubing. Dip catheter end into sterile water.

5. Gently thread the wet catheter into the tracheotomy tube.

6. Begin suctioning while slowly pulling the catheter out. Twirl the tube between the thumb and fore finger. Do not suction consecutively for more than 10 seconds since excessive removal of oxygen from the lungs can be dangerous.

7. Wait a minimum of 30 seconds to determine if an additional suctioning will be needed.

8. When finished suctioning, place the suction catheter tip back into the sterile water and remove any residue from catheter and tubing.

sterile water, bowl, and gloves (optional). Some sources recommend the use of saline solution instead of sterile water.

Even with the greatest of care and experience, unexpected situations arise that cannot be controlled in the home environment. A patient's caregiver should be trained in cardiopulmonary resuscitation, and be aware that alterations must be made to successfully resuscitate. The major difference is that mouth to mouth breathing is not effective and a mouth to stoma technique is required. The patient's airway is no longer closed through to the oral cavity and the tracheotomy site is now the primary site where breathing occurs. If respiratory distress occurs caregivers should initially establish an appropriate head tilt that allows easy access to the tracheotomy and opens the airway. A quick assessment of the patient's tracheotomy should be completed next, looking for mucus plugs or excessive secretions. If present, these secretions are then suctioned in an attempt to alleviate the situation. If problem breathing persists, attempt to change the tube. If no change in status, after replacing the tube, emergency services then must be contacted immediately as the situation is emergent. Manual ventilation then is started with a resuscitation bag. Normal resuscitation measures are implemented once an appropriate breathing pattern has been established. Caregivers must be educated to respond to situations urgently. They must be aware of signs of distress and how to intervene appropriately to solve the situation or when emergency services must be contacted. Caregivers may participate in mock scenarios to assist in preparing for true situations. It is suggested that caregivers have an emergency bag packed and readily available.

Patients should not attempt to limit themselves due to their tracheotomy. Although traveling long distances may be challenging, if one is organized it is definitely possible. A short day trip or overnight trip should be attempted initially to gain experience and confidence. Medical assistance should always be within a reasonable distance from your destination (don't go hiking in a remote, poorly accessible location with the nearest hospital 60 miles away) until the patient is medically stable, realistic of capabilities, and highly comfortable in managing their own tracheotomy.

When traveling, patients should pack enough supplies for the entire length of the trip along with a few additional supplies just to be prepared for unexpected delays. The list of supplies will vary depending on the needs and stability of the patient. The following is a list of basic supplies that will be needed. Some items may be obtained at the destination while others will have to be packed and travel with the patient.

- Portable suction machine – ideally two, and one may be obtained at the destination.
- Suction catheters.
- Portable oxygen – purchased at destination.
- Extra tracheotomy tubes of varying sizes.
- Gloves.
- Saline bullets.
- Scissors – these should be paramedic or blunt nose for traveling in the air.
- Medicine.
- Bulb syringe.
- Hand sanitizer.
- DeLee suction devices (for emergencies).
- List of emergency phone numbers.
- Emergency information card detailing medical condition.

Traveling on a plane requires the patient to make additional effort to be prepared. The airline must be informed in advance that special assistance will be needed. Airline security needs to be informed about special equipment that will be checked and that items need to remain clean and sterile. A letter from the patient's primary physician stating the medical necessity of the items and of any other medical conditions is helpful. This will give airline personnel an idea of what to look for and how to handle the equipment properly.

Simulation

If utilized properly, simulation can be a very effective method for teaching patients and caregivers, as well as professionals, the skills they will need to perform related to tracheotomy care. Mannequins called task trainers can be used to demonstrate and practice many of the techniques required for chronic care such as suctioning techniques, proper inflation, dressing changes, and other techniques such as stoma cleansing, changing tracheotomy tubes, and tube ties. The devices are available in adult, child, or infant sizes with anatomically correct oral and nasal passages, pharynx, epiglottis, esophagus, tracheotomy site, and cricoid cartilage as well as a right and left mainstem bronchial tree. Suctioning practice can be performed either via the tracheotomy or through the mouth or nose. Parents, caregivers, and patients can master techniques on the lifelike mannequin gaining the confidence needed to perform these tasks.

Several devices are made specifically for this purpose or other airway devices can often be modified to provide an adequate, but less expensive version. One mannequin made by Life/form (Mass Group Inc., Miami, FL, USA) is a tracheotomy care simulator set that comes complete with one adult and one infant mannequin, one adult and one infant tracheotomy tube, instruction guide, and hard carrying case for about $750–1000. This set is designed for professionals that perform and teach a high volume of patients about tracheotomies. A less expensive approach for suctioning education and training was developed by Patricia Pothier [2]. Her low-cost model can be built for less than $100.

Resources

There are many ways one can obtain training and education about tracheotomy care, but most agree that the best education comes from hands-on experience. As one gains experience, additional resources such as textbooks or journal articles, online information, videos, simulated learning via a mannequin, and advice and assistance of other patients and caregivers is helpful. Healthcare providers and caregivers can choose resources based on their preferred way of learning but appropriate learning resources can be challenging to find.

There is little doubt that patients and families experience significant stress, confusion, and frustration before, during, and after the placement of a tracheotomy. Typically, the sole burden of care is placed upon a close family member immediately following discharge from the hospital. This newfound responsibility coupled with somewhat limited written sources of information lead people to rely on support groups or knowledgeable providers to help teach, educate, and provide guidance. The Internet also provides individuals with easily accessible information and answers to basic questions without leaving their home or having to wait for a return phone call. Internet sites discussed on the following pages have been listed at the end of the chapter. One of the best known, most visible, and highly visited websites is called Aaron's Tracheostomy Page with the self-proclaimed title "The Internet's leading tracheostomy page" (www.tracheostomy.com). It has references, support group sites, a Facebook page, and a blog. This site demonstrates an interactive forum where people can ask questions and receive information from other individuals who have experienced similar situations. One thread for example is about bathing, showering, and even swimming with a tracheotomy in place. This site also has a vast number of links that assist individuals with equipment suppliers for both the general and specific needs.

An Internet search reveals many pamphlets, guides, and handouts from multiple academic institutions. The institutional publications typically provide general information pertaining to procedures and protocols at that specific site. There are cons to having an enormous quantity of information so readily available. One such difficulty is that rarely do different websites provide identical information. Caregivers and patients are then forced to filter through the information to determine which is the best and most reliable. The following table provides information regarding sites that have been deemed concise and accurate. Many of these sites were created strictly for personal use and have been written in a language specifically for caregivers and patients.

Support groups

Not all answers to questions can be found through the Internet or book. One philosophy subscribed to by professionals who focus on the direct care and teaching of tracheotomies is that the availability of a network of people in the same or similar situation is crucial to the newly tracheotomized patient. Therefore, tracheotomized patients and their primary caregivers are recommended to join support groups. It does not matter if an individual may go online or visit with friends in the community building. In the support group forums, a specific question may be posed and people from all over the country and even the world can talk about their experiences and knowledge as it pertains to the specific question posed.

Support groups are important to adult recovery as they allow adult patients the opportunity to meet other individuals experiencing the same emotions and stressors. Most communities have support groups that meet on a regular basis. There are multiple online

Table 14.6 Resources

http://www.tracheostomy.com/resources/pdf/University_Kentucky.pdf.	Eighteen page pamphlet, supplies the individual with information through multiple modalities, including pictures and lists of practical items Good for those who are new to tracheotomy care.
http://www.tracheostomy.com/resources/pdf/trachHandbk.pdf.	Fifty-two page guide directed specifically to healthcare providers, with a handbook titled *Tracheostomy Care Handbook* Created by Portex®, a maker of tracheotomy tubes and supplies.
http://www.thoracic.org/sections/education/care-of-the-child-with-a-chronic-tracheostomy	You will find many sections delineating specific criteria for completion of tasks and overall information. Includes clinical information education meetings, courses and publications.
www.lvnstudy.com/juniors/2009/10/31/tracheostomy-care-and-suction	Has videos that show patients, family, and caregivers, how to perform a tracheotomy intubation, and care for the endotracheal tube. There is also a tutorial on how to suction a tracheotomy tube and a blog on the left side of the screen.

Table 14.7 Books that focus on chronic care of the tracheotomy and/or stoma

(1) Meyers EN, Johnson JT. *Tracheotomy Airway Management, Communication, and Swallowing*, 2nd edn. San Diego, CA: Plural Publishing Inc. 2007.

(2) Dikeman KJ, Kazandjian MS. *Communication and Swallowing Management of Tracheostomized and Ventilator Dependent Adults*. New York: Singular, 2003.

(3) Tippett D. *Tracheostomy and Ventilator Dependency: Management of Breathing, Speaking, and Swallowing*. New York: Thieme, 2000.

(4) Adamo-Tumminelli P. *A Guide to Pediatric Tracheostomy Care (Plastic Comb)*, 2nd edition. Springfield, IL: Charles C. Thomas, 1993.

(5) Bissell CM. *Pediatric Tracheostomy Home Care Guide*. Sudbury, MA: Jones and Bartlett Learning, 2008.

support groups a patient may become involved with; however, most sites request that a patient posting discussion questions should pertain to tracheotomy care on some level.

Support group meetings are also available providing tracheotomized patients with the opportunity to meet people with similar experiences. Face-to-face interactions allow newly tracheotomized patients first-hand encounters with more experienced tracheotomy patients. The experienced tracheotomy patient can hand down wisdom that is only gained from trial and error, opportunities that the new patient has yet to encounter. "Brainstorming" during these meetings often leads patients to new funding sources and medical supplies they were unaware were available. Academic centers or large healthcare systems commonly have meetings for patients on a monthly basis. A patient may contact the oral maxillofacial or head and neck departments in their community or their surgeon, to inquire about meeting times for the local support group.

There are many online support groups. Yahoo has an online support group known as the "Neckbreathers." Their website is http://health.groups.yahoo.com/group/Neckbreathers. This group was founded in 2000 and consists of over 500 members. A patient must become a member of the group to have the resources available. Becoming a member provides the

Table 14.8 Best support groups

Neckbreathers	Great way for relatively new tracheotomy patients to get specific questions answered
Tracheotomy.info	Online community that offers a forum for discussion
Aaron's Tracheostomy page	Overall goal of the site is to promote mutual support and information sharing for persons who have or anticipate having a tracheotomy
Trachcare	To provide support and information to parents, caregivers, and healthcare providers of children who have, or previously had, a tracheotomy
Medela	Site for finding support groups for family and patient caregivers

opportunity to post questions or to respond to other's questions online. This is a great way for relatively new tracheotomy patients to get specific questions answered that were not initially thought of while in hospital.

Another useful Internet site is Tracheotomy.info found at www.tracheostomy.info and is an online community that offers a forum for discussion. According to the website, "it has been referred to by many folks around the world as the internet's leading destination for tracheostomy related information for adults and children." On this site, there are multiple discussion forums. News articles are posted pertaining to tracheotomy patients and there are over 300 (+) web links for items relating to tracheotomies.

Aaron's Tracheostomy Page was founded in 1998, by the mother of a child who had a tracheotomy for the first 4 years of his life. The overall goal of the site is to promote mutual support and information sharing for persons who have or anticipate having a tracheotomy. It is open to parents of children, patients, families, caregivers, and professionals. Aaron's Tracheostomy Page and web ring site is located at http://tracheostomy.com/ring/index.htm. The web ring aids users in quickly, easily, and reliably navigating thousands of related websites organized by areas of interest.

The internet address of Trachcare is http://www.trachcare.org/about.html. According to the site, "Trachcare" is a registered 501(c)(3) non-profit organization created to provide support and information to parents, caregivers, and healthcare providers of children who have, or previously had, a tracheotomy, and children who are on ventilator support. The site was founded in 2004 by parents in Massachusetts who have children with tracheotomies. This site is used for forums, or meetings with families will be organized to discuss specific topics relevant to the care of children with tracheotomies. The site also allows one to establish connection with other families, ways to cope with parenting challenges, identify resources available, and learn about training and conference opportunities.

One site for finding support groups for family and patient caregivers is www.medela.com/USA/suction/vacuumsystems/pumps/tracheostomy/clario_Refs.php.

Case conclusion

John went home from the rehabilitation facility. He requires 24-hour care provided by his wife, and homecare professionals. His wife was able to take medical leave from her work to stay at home with John. She had been trained in managing his tracheotomy; however, she was not confident with the independent implementation of techniques. She relied heavily on the home health nurse to assist in answering questions. Shortly after John was discharged home, he began to exhibit serious signs of depression. John's wife contacted their otolaryngologist-head and neck surgeon and social worker provided them with information to contact mental health professionals. With continued support from immediate family members, home healthcare professionals, and the addition of respite workers, a consistent routine was established. John and his family reached out to support groups in their area that provided additional information and techniques to assist with problem solving specific areas of trouble. Via therapists (speech, occupational, and physical) John was provided with equipment that allowed him to access the Internet. This permitted John to have the freedom to express his feelings, thoughts, and concerns via an anonymous outlet and to communicate with other tracheotomized patients.

Ultimately, after many months of rehabilitation, both physical and mental, John has been able to establish a functional pattern to his daily life. With constant effort, and the support of multiple individuals, both virtual and present, John has regained his ability to complete tasks he enjoyed before his accident.

References

1. Russell C, Matta B. *Tracheostomy: a Multiprofessional Handbook*. London: Greenwich Medical Media Limited, 2004; 296.

2. Pothier P. Low-cost tracheostomy model for suctioning simulation. *Nurs Educ* 2006; **31**(5): 192–4.

Internet resources

www.associatedcontent.com/article1520655/qualifying_for_home_health_care_services.html
www.beevers.net
www.calder.med.miami.edu/providers/SPEECH/speak.html
www.corporativonemedica.net
www.faculty.mercer.edu/summervill_j/jeanchiang/itisallaboutme.html
www.healthsquare.com
www.hopkinsmedicine.org/tracheostomy/living
www.MedScape.com
www.mycleavlandclinic.org/head_neck/patients/head_neck_cancer/tracheostomy_care.aspx
www.rainbowrehab.com/Rainbowvisionarticle_downloads/articles/Art-MED-Trach.pdf
www.rancho.org/patient%20education/selfcare
www.thoracic.org
www.tracheostomy.com
www.uwhealth.org
www.webwhispers.org/library/Postlaryngectomy.asp

Index

Aaron's Tracheostomy Page, 191
adenoid cystic carcinoma, 69
air dissection
  pediatric patients, 80
airway adjuncts, 51
airway manipulation with
    tracheotomy, 134–44
  apneic oxygenation, 144
  basic airway manipulation
    procedures, 135–7
  case scenario, 134
  case scenario outcome, 144
  complications, 137–8
  developments in advanced
    airway management, 134–5
  double lumen endotracheal
    tube, 139–40
  endobronchial blockade,
    140–3
  lung isolation, 138
  selective endobronchial
    intubation, 143–4
Allander, Claes, 169
American Association for
    Respiratory Care Clinical
    Practice Guidelines,
    168
American Society for Testing
    and Materials (ASTM)
    standards for tracheotomy
    tubes, 150
anatomic variations
  bronchogenic cysts, 65
  congenital high airway
    obstruction syndrome
    (CHAOS), 67–8
  congenital tracheal stenosis,
    66
  congenital tracheal webs, 66
  craniofacial syndromes
  embryology, 63
  esophageal anomalies, 65
  extrinsic airway obstruction,
    63–5
  goiter, 65
  infectious airway
    obstruction, 65
  infectious conditions, 68

inflammatory airway
    obstruction, 65
inflammatory conditions, 68
intrinsic airway obstruction,
    66–70
laryngeal clefts, 67
laryngeal webs, 67
laryngoesophageal clefts, 67
laryngomalacia, 67
laryngotracheal–esophageal
    clefts, 67
metabolic conditions, 68
nasal obstruction, 63–4
neoplasmic airway
    obstruction, 65
neoplastic disease, 69–70
oropharynx, 64
proliferative disease, 69–70
subglottic hemangiomas, 67
tracheal agenesis/atresia, 66
tracheomalacia, 66
trauma-related airway
    obstruction, 68–9
vascular anomalies, 64–5
vocal cord paralysis, 67
anatomy
  pediatric patients, 73–5
anatomy of the neck, 12–24
  arteries and veins, 14–17
  carotid sheath, 12–13
  cricoid cartilage, 20–1
  cricothyroid membrane, 21
  deep fascia, 12–13
  esophagus, 21–2
  fatty subcutaneous tissue, 12
  infrahyoid (strap) muscles, 14
  larynx, 20–1
  nerves of the central neck,
    18–19
  omohyoid muscle, 14
  placement of the
    tracheotomy, 23
  platysma muscle, 12
  pretracheal layer of the deep
    fascia, 12–13
  pretracheal space, 13–14
  prevertebral layer of the deep
    fascia, 12–13

relevance to tracheotomy,
    23–4
retroesophageal space, 13–14
retropharyngeal space, 13–14
retrovisceral space, 13–14
skin, 12
spaces and compartments
    below the hyoid bone,
    13–14
sternohyoid muscle, 14
sternothyroid muscle, 14
strap muscles, 14
superficial fascia, 12
superficial layer of the deep
    fascia, 12–13
thyrohyoid muscle, 14
thyroid cartilage, 20
thyroid gland, 19–20
trachea, 21–2
tracheal dimensions, 24
visceral compartment, 13
visceral structures of the
    neck, 19–22
ansa cervicalis, 18–19
anterior cricoid split
    procedure, 91
anterior jugular vein, 17
apneic oxygenation, 144
Arndt bronchial blocker
    (Cook), 140
arteries and veins, 14–17
  anterior jugular vein, 17
  arteries of the central
    neck, 16
  carotid bifurcation, 16
  carotid sheath, 16
  common carotid artery, 16
  deep veins of the central
    neck, 17
  external carotid artery and
    branches, 16
  external jugular vein, 17
  inferior thyroid artery, 15–16
  innominate artery, 15
  internal carotid artery, 16
  internal jugular vein, 17
  subclavian artery and
    branches, 14–16

arteries and veins (cont.)
superficial veins of the central neck, 17
suprascapular (transverse scapular) artery, 15, 16
thyrocervical trunk, 15–16
thyroid ima artery, 19
tracheoinnominate artery erosion, 15
transverse cervical artery, 15, 16
vertebral artery, 15
aspiration, 120, 131–2
Assist Control, 136
asthma, 166
atherosclerosis, 22

bacterial tracheitis, 68
bath trachs, 184–5
bilateral vocal cord paralysis, 29, 40, 67
Bivonna tracheotomy tube, 136
Björk flap, 32
blade incision
cricothyroidotomy, 55–6
bleeding
after tracheotomy, 118–19
operatively or postoperatively, 34
brachiocephalic (innominate) trunk, 14
brain injury
timing of tracheotomy, 102–3
bronchial carcinoid, 69
bronchogenic cysts, 65
bronchotomy, 4
bubble humidifier, 168
burn injury, 29

can't ventilate can't intubate (CVCI) emergency
cardiopulmonary resuscitation training for carers, 189
cardiothoracic surgery patients
mediastinitis risk with tracheotomy, 106–7
use of tracheotomy, 105–6
carotid bifurcation, 16
carotid sinus, 16
cellulitis, 81
choanal atresia, 63–4
CHARGE syndrome, 63–4
chronic obstruction pulmonary disease, 22, 166
chronic obstructive lung disease, 8

chronically ill patients
use of tracheotomy, 108–9
Ciaglia method (percutaneous dilating technique), 41–2
common carotid artery, 16
complications of tracheotomy, 34–6, 126–32
after percutaneous tracheotomy, 48–9
aspiration, 120, 131–2
bleeding, 34, 118–19
case presentation, 126
case resolution, 132
dislodgement of the tracheal tube, 119
early complications, 118–20
erosion caused by the tracheal tube, 132
foreign body in tracheal tube or airway, 127–8
granulation tissue, 34
hemorrhage, 34, 118, 129–30
hypotension, 120
ICU patients, 118–19
inadvertent decannulation, 34–5
infection, 35, 131
inflammation, 131
late complications
loss of airway with tracheal tube removal, 128–9
major complication rate in ICU patients, 118
malnutrition, 131–2
mucosal irritation, 131
nosocomial pneumonia
obstruction of the tracheotomy tube, 119
pearls, 132
percutaneous dilation tracheotomy, 131
pneumomediastinum, 35
pneumonitis, 131–2
pneumothorax, 35, 119
postoperative hemorrhage, 129–30
scarring, 131
subcutaneous emphysema, 120, 131
swallowing dysfunction, 131–2
thyroid laceration, 120
tracheal cuff complications, 119
tracheal stenosis, 35–6, 131

tracheal tube obstruction, 126–7
tracheoesophageal fistula, 22, 36, 128
tracheoesophageal perforation, 120
tracheoinnominate artery erosion, 15
tracheoinnominate artery fistula, 36, 118–19
tracheomalacia, 36
tube displacement, 119
tube obstruction, 34
congenital anomalies
embryology, 63
congenital high airway obstruction syndrome (CHAOS)
ex utero intrapartum treatment (EXIT), 67–8
congenital tracheal stenosis, 66
congenital tracheal webs, 66
Cook Ardt bronchial blocker, 140
Cook Percutaneous Tracheostomy Introducer Set, 163
craniofacial syndromes
associated airway anomalies
craniomaxillofacial trauma
use of tracheotomy, 104–5
cricoid cartilage, 20–1
cricothyroid membrane, 21
cricothyroidotomy
cricothyroid membrane, 21
See also emergency cricothyroidotomy.
cricotracheal resection procedure, 92–3
croup, 3, 68
cutaneous innervation, 18
cynanche trachealis, 3
cystic fibrosis, 166

decannulation
accidental (pediatric patients), 82
inadvertent, 34–5
planned, 34
planned (pediatric), 84
unwanted closure of the tracheotomy site, 136
deep fascia, 12–13
Dick, Elisha Cullen, 1, 4, 9
dilation over guidewire techniques, 39

diphtheria, 2, 6, 29, 72
dornase alfa, 166
double lumen endotracheal
    tube
    airway manipulation, 139–40
dysphagia, 182–3
    pediatric tracheotomy
        patients, 81
    See also swallowing
        dysfunction

eating difficulty
    swallow evaluation, 182–3
elderly patients
    use of tracheotomy, 108–9
elective surgical tracheotomy
    (adult), 28–36
    Björk flap, 32
    clinical scenario, 28
    complications, 34–6
    contraindications, 29
    decannulation, 34
    definition of tracheotomy, 28
    indications, 28–9
    operative technique, 30–3
    patient groups who may
        benefit, 28
    postoperative care, 34
    potential benefits for
        patients, 28
    preoperative evaluation, 29
    tracheal window, 32
    tracheotomy tube selection,
        33–4
    types of tracheal incision, 32
    vertical tracheal incision, 32
embryology
    congenital anomalies, 63
emergency cricothyroidotomy,
    51–60
    anatomy, 52–3
    blade incision techniques,
        55–6
    can't ventilate can't intubate
        (CVCI) emergency
        case study, 51, 60, 70–
    classification of
        cricothyroidotomy
        techniques, 53
    complications, 57–8
    contraindications, 53
    cost, 59
    efficacy of ventilation, 59
    experience and choice of
        technique, 59
    history of development, 52

indications, 53
jet ventilators, 54–5
needle puncture
    techniques, 53
post-cricothyroidotomy
    management, 59
recommendations, 58–9
risk of trauma, 59
situational considerations, 58
speed of insertion, 58
surgical cricothyroidotomy,
    55–6
techniques, 54
training methods, 59–60
use of animal preparations
    for training, 60
use of cadavers for training,
    60
use of mannequins for
    training, 60
endobronchial blockade, 140–3
endotracheal intubation, 6
eosinophilic esophagitis, 88
epiglottitis, 29
erosion caused by the tracheal
    tube, 132
esophageal anomalies, 65
esophagus
    gross anatomy, 21–2
ex utero intrapartum treatment
    (EXIT), 67–8
expectorants, 167
external carotid artery and
    branches, 16
external jugular vein, 17

facial trauma
    use of tracheotomy,
        104–5
Fantoni's technique
    (translaryngeal approach),
        45–7
fenestrated tracheotomy tubes,
    156–7
fiberoptic bronchoscopy, 137
fiberoptic endoscopic
    examination of swallowing
    (FEES), 182
flexible laryngobronchoscopy,
    89
Fogarty embolectomy
    catheters, 140
foreign body in tracheal tube or
    airway, 127–8
French sizing system
    tracheotomy tubes, 151

gastric tube (G tube), 183
gastroesophageal reflux
    (GERD), 88
Glide-Scope (Verathon
    Medical), 51
goiter
    airway obstruction, 65
granulation tissue, 34, 175–6
granuloma formation
    pediatric tracheotomy, 82
Griggs technique (guidewire
    dilating forceps
    technique), 43–5
guidewire dilating forceps
    (GWDF) development, 9
guidewire dilating forceps
    technique (Griggs
    technique), 43–5

heat and moisture exchange
    (HME) devices, 169–70
heated humidifier systems
    (HHS), 168–9
hemangioma, 69
hemorrhage
    after tracheotomy, 118
    complication of
        tracheotomy, 34
    pediatric patients, 80, 81
    postoperative, 129–30
high spinal cord injury (SCI)
    timing of tracheotomy,
        101–2
history of tracheotomy, 1–9
    advent of antibiotics, 6
    Albucasis, 2
    Alexander the Great, 1
    ancient Egypt, 1
    ancient Hindu medicine, 1
    Aretaeus, 1
    Asclepiades of Bithynia,
        1–2
    bronchotomy, 4
    changing terminology, 4
    development of guide wire
        dilating forceps (GWDF), 9
    development of
        percutaneous dilational
        tracheotomy, 9
    Ebers Papyrus, 1
    Homer, 1
    improvements in tube
        design, 4–5, 8
    laryngotomy, 4
    period of dramatization
        (AD 1833), 4–6

history of tracheotomy (cont.)
  period of enthusiasm
    (AD 1932), 8
  period of fear (AD 1546), 2–4
  period of legend (3100 BC to
    AD 1546), 1–2
  period of rationalization (AD
    1965 to the present), 8–9
  Seldinger technique, 9
  use for laryngeal abscess, 2
  use in intensive care, 8
  use in poliomyelitis, 8
  use in war wound
    management, 6, 8
  work of Chevalier Jackson,
    4–5
home care of tracheotomy,
    180–94
  bath trachs, 184–5
  cardiopulmonary
    resuscitation training for
    carers, 189
  case presentation, 180,
    182–3, 193–4
  difficulty eating, 182–3
  discharge planning, 181
  emergency situations, 189
  equipment required, 183–5
  home health providers, 181
  humidification collar, 184
  Internet resources, 191–3
  multidisciplinary support
    team, 180–3
  patient and caregiver
    guidelines, 186–93
  plan for possible
    decannulation, 181
  resources for education,
    training and support, 191–3
  respite workers, 181
  role of the physician, 181
  role of the social
    worker, 181
  role of the speech language
    pathologist, 181–3
  shower shields, 184–5
  simulation training, 190
  skills required, 180
  speaking valves, 181–2, 183
  stoma shields, 184
  suctioning, 188–9
  support for tracheotomy
    patients, 180–3
  support groups, 193–4
  swallow evaluation, 182–3
  swimming, 184–5

tracheotomy education for
    patients, 180–3
  tracheotomy guards, 184
  training for emergencies, 189
  traveling arrangements,
    189–90
  typical cleaning instructions,
    186–8
home health providers
  home care of tracheotomy, 181
humidification, 167–71
  bubble humidifier, 168
  heat and moisture exchange
    (HME) devices, 169–70
  heated humidifier systems
    (HHS), 168–9
  methods to humidify air,
    168–71
  normal heat and moisture
    exchange, 167–8
  passover humidifier, 168
humidification collar, 184
Hunter syndrome, 68
hypertonic saline therapy, 167
hypoglossal nerve, 18–19
hypotension
  tracheotomy complication,
    120

iatrogenic trauma
  pediatric patients, 80
ICU tracheal care, 117–19
  aspiration, 120
  bleeding after tracheotomy,
    118–19
  case presentation, 117
  complications of
    tracheotomy, 118–19
  dislodgement of the tracheal
    tube, 119
  early complications of
    tracheotomy, 118–20
  early tracheotomy, 122
  hemorrhage after
    tracheotomy, 118
  hypotension, 120
  indications for tracheotomy,
    117
  infection
  late complications of
    tracheotomy
  management of minor
    bleeds, 118–19
  nosocomial pneumonia
  objectives of tracheotomy
    care, 120

obstruction of the
    tracheotomy tube, 119
  open surgical tracheotomy,
    117–18
  oxygen desaturation, 120
  patient comfort, 120
  percutaneous dilational
    tracheotomy, 117–18
  pneumothorax, 119
  potential benefits of early
    tracheotomy, 122
  protocol for tracheotomy
    care, 120
  subcutaneous emphysema,
    120
  thyroid laceration, 120
  timing of tracheotomy, 118,
    122
  tracheal cuff complications,
    119
  tracheal stenosis
  tracheoesophageal fistula
  tracheoesophageal
    perforation, 120
  tracheoinnominate artery
    fistula
  tracheotomy techniques,
    117–18
  tracheotomy tube selection,
    119
  tube displacement, 119
  typical tracheotomy care
    procedures, 120
  weaning from mechanical
    ventilation, 122
  weaning from tracheotomy,
    122
indications for tracheotomy,
    28–9, 39–40, 117
infection
  airway obstruction, 65, 68
  complication of
    tracheotomy, 35, 131
  pediatric tracheotomy, 81
inferior thyroid artery,
    15–16
inflammation following
    tracheotomy, 131
inflammatory airway
    obstruction, 65
inflammatory conditions, 68
infrahyoid (strap) muscles, 14
initial care of tracheotomy,
    165–78
  case presentation, 165
  case resolution, 000

challenges faced by
  tracheotomy patients, 165
composition of mucus, 166
expectorants, 167
failure of the tracheotomy
  tube, 177
granulation tissue, 175–6
humidification, 167–71
hypertonic saline therapy,
  167
initial tube exchange, 174–5
key issues, 178
monitoring tracheotomy
  tube function, 177
mucokinetic agents, 167
mucolytics, 167
mucoregulators, 167
mucus, 166
N-acetylcysteine therapy, 167
normal heat and moisture
  exchange, 167–8
normal saline installation,
  173–4
properties of mucus, 166
routine changes of
  tracheotomy tube, 177
secretion removal, 167
secretions, 166
sputum, 166
sterile versus clean
  technique, 174
suctioning, 171–3
swallowing dysfunction, 167
thin and copious secretions,
  167
wound care and cleaning,
  176–7
wound management,
  174–7
innominate (brachiocephalic)
  trunk, 14
innominate artery
  erosion by a tracheotomy
    tube, 15
  high riding, 30
  tracheoinnominate artery
    fistula, 36
internal carotid artery, 16
internal jugular vein, 17
International Standards
  Organization (ISO)
  sizing of tracheotomy tubes,
    151
Internet
  resources for tracheotomy
    patients, 191–3

intubated patients. *See* timing
  of tracheotomy for
  intubated patients
isothermal saturation point or
  boundary (ISB), 167

Jackson, Chevalier, 4–5
jet ventilators, 54–5

Langer's lines, 12
laryngeal clefts, 67
laryngeal edema, 29
laryngeal mask airways (LMA),
  51, 138
laryngeal webs, 67
laryngoesophageal clefts, 67
laryngomalacia, 67
laryngotomy, 4
laryngotracheal reconstruction,
  87–95
  analgesia for pediatric
    patients, 90–1
  anesthetic management for
    pediatric patients, 89–91
  anterior cricoid split, 91
  cricotracheal resection, 92–3
  double-stage approach, 88
  endoscopic treatment, 91
  flexible
    laryngobronchoscopy, 89
  intraoperative management,
    89–93
  laryngotracheoplasty with
    cartilage grafting, 91–2
  pediatric case 1, 87
  pediatric case 2, 87
  postoperative considerations
    for pediatric patients, 94–5
  postoperative stenting, 88
  preoperative considerations
    in pediatric patients,
    88–9
  rigid direct laryngoscopy and
    bronchoscopy, 89
  single-stage approach, 88
  subglottic stenosis grading
    scale, 87
  surgical management, 91–3
  timing considerations, 88–9
  types of open airway
    procedures, 87–8
laryngotracheal–esophageal
  clefts, 67
laryngotracheobronchitis, 68
laryngotracheoplasty with
  cartilage grafting, 91–2

larynx
  anatomy, 20–1
  cricoid cartilage, 20–1
  thyroid cartilage, 20
low profile tracheotomy tubes,
  157
Ludwig's angina, 2, 29
lung isolation, 138

malnutrition
  complication of
    tracheotomy, 131–2
Martin, George, 4
maxillofacial trauma, 29
median sternotomy
  mediastinitis risk with
    tracheotomy, 106–7
mediastinitis
  complication of tracheotomy
    risk with tracheotomy, 106–7
metabolic conditions, 68
modified barium swallow study
  (MBSS), 182, 183
Montgomery tracheal
  T-tube, 158
MUC genes, 166
MUC5AC gene, 166
mucokinetic agents, 167
mucolytics, 167
mucoregulators, 167
mucosal irritation, 131
mucus, 166
  composition, 166
  functions, 166
  MUC genes, 166
  properties, 166
multidisciplinary support team,
  180–3
multiple trauma
  timing of tracheotomy,
    103–4
mumps, 2
myasthenia gravis, 8

N-acetylcysteine therapy, 167
nasal obstruction
  congenital, 63–4
needle puncture
  cricothyroidotomy, 53
neoplasm
  airway obstruction, 65
neoplastic disease, 69–70
nerves of the central neck,
  18–19
  ansa cervicalis, 18–19
  cutaneous innervation, 18

nerves of the central neck (cont.)
  hypoglossal nerve, 18–19
  tenth nerve and its
    branches, 18
  twelfth nerve, 18–19
  vagus nerve and its
    branches, 18
nosocomial pneumonia
Nu-trach (Portex), 137

omohyoid muscle, 14
open surgical tracheotomy,
    117–18
oral or oropharyngeal
    tumors, 29
oropharynx, 64
oxygen desaturation
    tracheotomy complication,
    120

palliative use of tracheotomy, 4
papillomatosis, 69
passover humidifier, 168
Passy–Muir valve, 28, 182, 183
patient education. *See* home
    care of tracheotomy
pediatric airway stenosis. *See*
    laryngotracheal
    reconstruction
pediatric patients
  percutaneous tracheotomy, 40
pediatric tracheotomy, 72–85
  anatomy, 73–5
  anesthetic management of
    tracheotomy, 78–9
  decannulation (planned), 84
  decision to perform
    tracheostomy, 72–3
  history of the procedure, 72
  home care, 79
  indications for, 72, 109
  mortality, 84–5
  outcomes, 84–5
  post-operative care, 77
  pre-operative evaluation, 73
  speech and language
    development difficulties, 85
  surveillance, 79–80
  technique, 75–7
  timing of tracheotomy in
    trauma patients, 111–12
  timing of, 110–11
  See also anatomic variations
pediatric tracheotomy
    complications
  accidental decannulation, 82

air dissection, 80
cellulitis, 81
dysphagia, 81
early postoperative
    complications, 81–2
granuloma formation, 82
hemorrhage (early
    postoperative), 81
hemorrhage (intraoperative),
    80
iatrogenic trauma, 80
intraoperative
    complications, 80–1
late postoperative
    complications, 82–4
obstruction of the
    tracheotomy tube, 81–2
persistent tracheocutaneous
    fistula, 83–4
pneumonia, 81
postobstructive pulmonary
    edema, 81
subglottic stenosis, 83
suprastomal collapse, 82–3
tracheal stenosis, 83
tracheitis, 81
tracheoesophageal fistula, 83
tracheoinnominate artery
    fistula, 83
tracheotomy tube problems,
    80–1
wound infection, 81
pediatric trauma patients
  timing of tracheotomy,
    111–12
PercTwist (screw-action
    dilator), 47
percutaneous dilational
    tracheotomy, 117–18
  complications, 131
  development, 9
percutaneous tracheotomy,
    39–49
  anesthesia considerations,
    47–8
  anesthetic considerations,
    40
  Ciaglia method
    (percutaneous dilating
    technique), 41–2
  contraindications, 40
  cost, 39
  development of the
    approach, 39
  dilation over guide wire
    techniques, 39

Fantoni's technique
    (translaryngeal approach),
    45–7
Griggs technique (guidewire
    dilating forceps
    technique), 43–5
indications, 39–40
limitations, 40
pediatric patients, 40
PercTwist (screw-action
    dilator), 47
postoperative complications,
    48–9
potential benefits for
    patients, 40
preoperative workup, 40
Seldinger technique, 39, 40
techniques, 40–7
time required, 39
percutaneous tracheotomy
    tubes, 161–3
persistent tracheocutaneous
    fistula, 83–4
Phonate speaking valve, 182
platysma muscle, 12
pneumomediastinum, 35
pneumonia, 8
  nosocomial, 000
  pediatric patients, 81
pneumonitis, 131–2
pneumothorax, 35, 119
poliomyelitis, 29
postobstructive pulmonary
    edema, 81
post-tracheotomy care and
    management
  team approach, 109
premeasured suctioning, 188
pretracheal space, 13–14
proliferative disease, 69–70

recurrent laryngeal nerves, 31
relapsing polychondritis, 68
respite workers
  home care of tracheotomy,
    181
retroesophageal space, 13–14
retropharyngeal space, 13–14
retrovisceral space, 13–14
rigid direct laryngoscopy and
    bronchoscopy, 89

scarring following
    tracheotomy, 131
screw-action dilators
  PercTwist, 47

secretion removal
    initial care of tracheotomy,
    167
Seldinger technique, 9, 39, 40,
    53
selective endobronchial
    intubation, 143–4
Shikani French speaking valve,
    182
Shiley PERC tracheotomy tube,
    163
shower shields, 184–5
simulation training
    for home care of
    tracheotomy, 190
sleep apnea, 64
sleep apnea prophylaxis, 40
social worker
    support role, 181
speaking tracheotomy tubes,
    159–60
speaking valves, 135, 160–1,
    181–2, 183
speech language pathologist,
    181–3
spinal cord injury (SCI)
    timing of tracheotomy, 101–2
sputum, 166
squamous cell carcinoma, 69
sterile versus clean technique
    initial care of tracheotomy,
    174
sternohyoid muscle, 14
sternothyroid muscle, 14
stoma shields, 184
strap muscles, 14
subclavian artery and branches,
    14–16
subcutaneous emphysema, 120,
    131
subglottic hemangiomas, 67
subglottic stenosis, 72
    pediatric tracheotomy
    patient, 83
    See also laryngotracheal
    reconstruction
suctioning
    deep suctioning, 188
    home care of tracheotomy,
    188–9
    initial care of tracheotomy,
    171–3
    open versus closed
    suctioning systems, 172–3
    premeasured, 188
    risks of suctioning, 171–2

shallow suctioning, 188
support groups for
    tracheotomy patients,
    191–3
supraglottoplasty, 67
suprascapular (transverse
    scapular) artery, 15, 16
suprastomal collapse
    pediatric tracheotomy, 82–3
swallow evaluation, 182–3
swallowing dysfunction, 131–2,
    167
    See also dysphagia
swimming with a tracheotomy,
    184–5
Synchronous Intermittent
    Mandatory Ventilation,
    136

team approach to post-
    tracheotomy care, 109
tenth nerve and its branches, 18
tetanus, 8, 29
thyrocervical trunk, 15–16
thyrohyoid muscle, 14
thyroid cartilage, 20
thyroid gland
    anatomy, 19–20
thyroid ima artery, 19, 31
thyroid laceration, 120
tight to shaft tracheotomy
    tubes, 154
timing of laryngotracheal
    reconstruction, 88–9
timing of tracheotomy
    craniomaxillofacial trauma,
    104–5
    facial trauma, 104–5
    ICU patients, 118, 122
    pediatric patients, 110–11
    pediatric trauma patients,
    111–12
timing of tracheotomy for
    intubated patients
    brain injury, 102–3
    cardiothoracic surgery
    patients, 105–6
    case presentation, 99
    case resolution, 112–13
    chronically ill patients, 108–9
    elderly patients, 108–9
    elective tracheotomy in the
    ICU, 99–101
    high spinal cord injury (SCI),
    101–2
    multiple trauma, 103–4

potential benefits for
    patients, 99–101, 107–8
trauma not involving the
    CNS, 103–4
traumatic brain injury,
    102–3
total laryngectomy, 136
trachea, 21–2
    dimensions in children and
    adults, 24
    gross anatomy, 21–2
    histology, 21
    innervation, 21
    lymphatics, 21
    vascular supply, 21
tracheal agenesis/atresia, 66
tracheal buttons, 158
tracheal cuff complications, 119
tracheal incision
    types of, 32
tracheal stenosis
    after tracheotomy, 131
    complication of
    tracheotomy, 35–6
    congenital, 66
    pediatric tracheotomy
    patient, 83
tracheal webs
    congenital, 66
tracheal window, 32
tracheitis, 81
tracheobronchomalacia, 64
tracheocutaneous fistula, 83–4
tracheoesophageal fistula, 22,
    36, 83, 128
tracheoesophageal perforation,
    120
tracheoinnominate artery
    erosion, 15
tracheoinnominate artery
    fistula, 36, 118–19
    pediatric patient, 83
tracheomalacia, 65, 66
    complication of
    tracheotomy, 36
tracheotomy equipment
    case presentation, 146
    case report outcome, 163
    current controversies,
    149–50
    functional components of a
    tracheotomy tube, 146–9
    special considerations,
    149–50
tracheotomy guards, 184
tracheotomy placement

tracheotomy placement (cont.)
and neck anatomy, 23
tracheotomy teams
post-tracheotomy care, 109
tracheotomy tube obstruction, 34
tracheotomy tubes
construction materials, 150–1
cuffless tubes, 147–8
current controversies, 149–50
dimensions, 33–4
dual cannula versus single cannula, 151
extra length tubes, 153
failure of, 177
fenestrated tracheotomy tubes, 156–7
fixing in place, 149
flange, 148–9
functional components, 146–9
inflatable cuff, 146–8
inner cannula, 146
low profile tracheotomy tubes, 157
monitoring tube function, 177
Montgomery tracheal T-tube, 158
obturator, 146
outer cannula, 146
percutaneous tracheotomy tubes, 161–3
proportions, 151–6
routine changes, 177

selection, 24, 33–4, 119, 153–6
sizes, 151–6
sizing systems, 151–3
speaking tracheotomy tubes, 159–60
speaking valves, 160–1
special considerations, 149–50
special purpose tubes and accessories, 157–63
standards, 150–1
tight to shaft type, 154
tracheal buttons, 158
types, 33–4
typical sizes for women and men, 154
with subglottic suction ports, 159
translaryngeal airways
long-term complications, 28–9
translaryngeal approach (Fantoni's technique), 45–7
transverse cervical artery, 15, 16
trauma not involving the central nervous system
timing of tracheotomy, 103–4
trauma-related airway obstruction, 68–9
traumatic brain injury
timing of tracheotomy, 102–3
traveling arrangements
tracheotomy patients, 189–90

trisomy 18, 65
trisomy 21, 65
Trousseau dilator, 55
twelfth nerve, 18–19

UniPerc (Portex), 161
Univent endotracheal tube, 140
upper airway tumors, 29

vagus nerve and its branches, 18
vascular anomalies, 64–5
VATER/VACTERL anomalies, 65
veins. *See* arteries and veins
ventilator-associated pneumonia (VAP), 108, 173
ventilator-dependent respiratory failure, 72
vertebral artery, 15
video laryngoscopes, 51
visceral compartment, 13
visceral structures of the neck, 19–22
vocal cord paralysis, 67

Washington, George, 1, 4, 9
weaning from mechanical ventilation, 122
weaning from tracheotomy, 122
wound care and cleaning, 176–7
wound infection
pediatric patients, 81
wound management, 174–7